BIOLOGY OF MYELOMONOCYTIC CELLS

Edited by **Anirban Ghosh**

Biology of Myelomonocytic Cells
http://dx.doi.org/10.5772/63122
Edited by Anirban Ghosh

Contributors

Luciana Marti, Nydia Bacal, Laiz Cameirão, Fernanda Rocha, Andrés Castell, Gabriela Piñón-Zárate, Miguel Herrera-Enríquez, Katia Jarquín-Yáñez, Iliana Medina-Solares, Haijun Li, Zhengkun Tu, Jiyu Li, Yuanyuan Ma, Muqing Yang, Zhigang He, Kenneth McCullough, Rajni Sharma, Brian Wigdahl, Michael Nonnemacher, Vanessa Pirrone, Shane Quiterio, Alexander Allen, Anthony Mele

Published by InTech

Janeza Trdine 9, 51000 Rijeka, Croatia

Publishing Process Manager Romina Rovan
Technical Editor SPi Global
Cover InTech Design team

First published May, 2017
Printed in Croatia
Legal deposit, Croatia: National and University Library in Zagreb

Additional hard copies can be obtained from orders@intechopen.com

Biology of Myelomonocytic Cells, Edited by Anirban Ghosh
p. cm.
Print ISBN 978-953-51-3123-6
Online ISBN 978-953-51-3124-3

For EU product safety concerns:
IN TECH d.o.o., Prolaz Marije Krucifikse Kozulić 3, 51000 Rijeka, Croatia,
info@intechopen.com or visit our website at intechopen.com.

Meet the editor

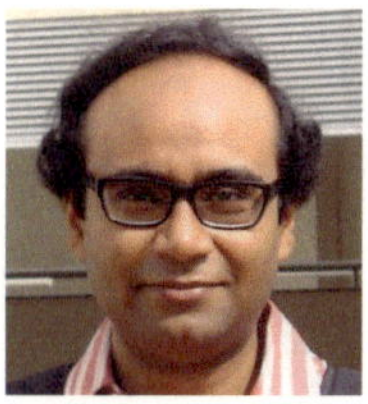

Dr. Anirban Ghosh completed his PhD degree from Calcutta University with the fellowship from Council of Scientific and Industrial Research (CSIR), India, in 2006 on the role of brain macrophage/microglia in glioma. Since then, with teaching, he has been pursuing research over a decade on brain macrophage and microglia in the development and disease as well as on basic glioma biology. His research is supported by multiple prominent funding agencies like UGC, SERB, CSIR, ICMR, etc. of the Indian Government. Dr. Ghosh has over 30 research articles in various journals and books; he is the recipient of various fellowships, medals and awards; an editorial board member and a reviewer of various journals; and an editor of book and journal volumes of international repute.

Contents

Preface

Myelomonocytes are the multipotent cells in the stage of blood cell differentiation, which are capable of generating the so-called innate components of immunity. Mainly comprising blood monocytes, tissue macrophages and subset of dendritic cells, this lineage actually serves as the evolutionary primitive arm of immunity. But these cells are those that reach almost every corner of our body including the restricted brain compartment, reside there as the guard, engage in constant surveillance in the territories and convey the health bulletin. Actually, their position and ability of judgement of the health of tissue or organ environment are the key initiators of tissue-specific immune response in a local and global fashion. Interestingly, the morpho-functional aspects of this group of cells vary to a wide range with their positional diversity. Their differentiation status, dynamics of lineage commitment, receptor expression and modulation and morphological and immune responses are now showing us various critical versatility, diversions or overlaps during differentiation and/or diseases. Therefore, understanding their biology is becoming crucial to know the tissue-specific immune activities and their modulation in normal physiological and patho-physiological situations. Their ability to communicate or represent the tissue microenvironment to the peripheral immune system and efficiency to engage the system to effector activation, modulation, support, and control hold the key for a successful immune endeavour. The present volume shows some glimpses of such an extensive area of current research interest of present immunology research.

'Biology' is a term that possesses the inherent power of inclusion that vortexes into all morphological, structural and functional aspects of a living entity. When the name of the present book volume was proposed, it was targeted to include the wide variation in terms of lineage divergence of the myelomonocytic precursor cells, their residential status in different parts of our body and their functional versatility as defender and effecter immune cell. As the editor of this volume, I expected wider participation and broader magnitude to cover, particularly, for the differentiated tissue resident myelomonocytic lineage cells. However, this is qualitatively compensated by the existing articles that precisely and efficiently deal with some very important, critical and timely aspects of myelomonocytic lineage cell biology and its challenging facets. The volume contains some articles that address some basic aspects of lineage differentiation of dendritic cells and few deal with morpho-functional aspects of these cells in organs and in diseases. The book is divided into two sections. The first section title is 'Lineage, Identity and Function', under which the article of Dr. Marti Luciana and colleagues deals with the lineage-specific and differentiation markers, their expression profile and their functional correlation to identify and characterize differentiating myelomonocytic cells, whereas the second one by Dr. Castell Andres and his colleagues discusses about variable precursors and lineages of dendritic cells, their characters, their functions and other immunological aspects. The second section of the book 'Function in Organ and Disease' comprises four chapters. The first chapter of this section by Prof Li and colleagues discusses about resident myelomonocytic cell in liver diseases; the second one by Dr. Li and Tu states the role of monocyte/macrophage in viral hepatitis, whereas the next one by Dr. McCullough and Sharma establishes the functional importance of dendritic cell endocytosis. Finally, Prof. Wigdhal and team demonstrate a newer application of myelomonocytic cell lines in virus-induced immunodeficiency disease modelling.

It was an interesting task that I initiated with the proposal from InTech last year. Though it is not a huge volume, it took a lengthy tenure partly because of the repeated editorial demand to the authors for more precision and largely because of several deadlines missed by me as an editor to complete the steps due to my several preoccupancies. Throughout the period, the support team of InTech and particularly Publishing Process Manager Ms. Romina Rovan cooperated with me a lot and managed to maintain all particulars to complete the book. I am thankful to them. I would also like to acknowledge the support of many who inspired me as an advisor, a supporter or a colleague and helped me as a student or staff at any time during this work. Lastly and most importantly, I would like to thank my family, my wife Malabika and my son Upamanyu for their presence, support and tolerance to my continuous involvement in the present work and many others throughout the time. This effort will be successful if the volume can add something in the understanding and research on myelomonocytic cells.

Anirban Ghosh
Panihati Mahavidyalaya,
Sodepur, India

Section 1

Lineage, Identity and Function

Chapter 1

Phenotypic Markers and Functional Regulators of Myelomonocytic Cells

Luciana Cavalheiro Marti, Nydia Strachman Bacal, Laiz Camerão Bento and Fernanda Agostini Rocha

Additional information is available at the end of the chapter

http://dx.doi.org/10.5772/67324

Abstract

In this chapter, there is a description of hematopoietic stem cells, maturation curve and their differentiation into myeloid cells, including phenotypes and transcription factors involved in this process. Further, we discuss myeloid maturation curve from myeloid precursor, monoblast, premonocyte to monocytes, and also monocytes subsets regarding their CD14 and CD16 expressions and related functions in health and disease. In addition, we reason about the differentiation from monocytes either in dendritic cells or in macrophages *in vitro* using differential growth factors; these cells are differentiated from those found *in vivo* being named as monocyte-derived cells. Furthermore, we explore distinguished phenotype of monocytes, macrophages, and dendritic cells monocyte-derived *in vitro*, using confocal microscopy and flow cytometry, in order to display morphological and phenotypic differences among them.

Keywords: myelomonocytic cells, monoblast, promonocytes, dendritic cells, monocytes

1. Introduction

All the cellular elements of blood derive ultimately from the hematopoietic stem cells in the bone marrow. Thus, the blood cells are derived from the common lymphoid progenitor and the myeloid progenitor, apart from the megakaryocytes and red blood cells that are derived from specific progenitors. Particularly, the lymphoid progenitor gives rise to natural killer (NK) cells, T and B lineage cells of the human immune system, while the myeloid progenitor is the precursor of the granulocytes, monocytes, macrophages, and dendritic cells (**Figure 1**).

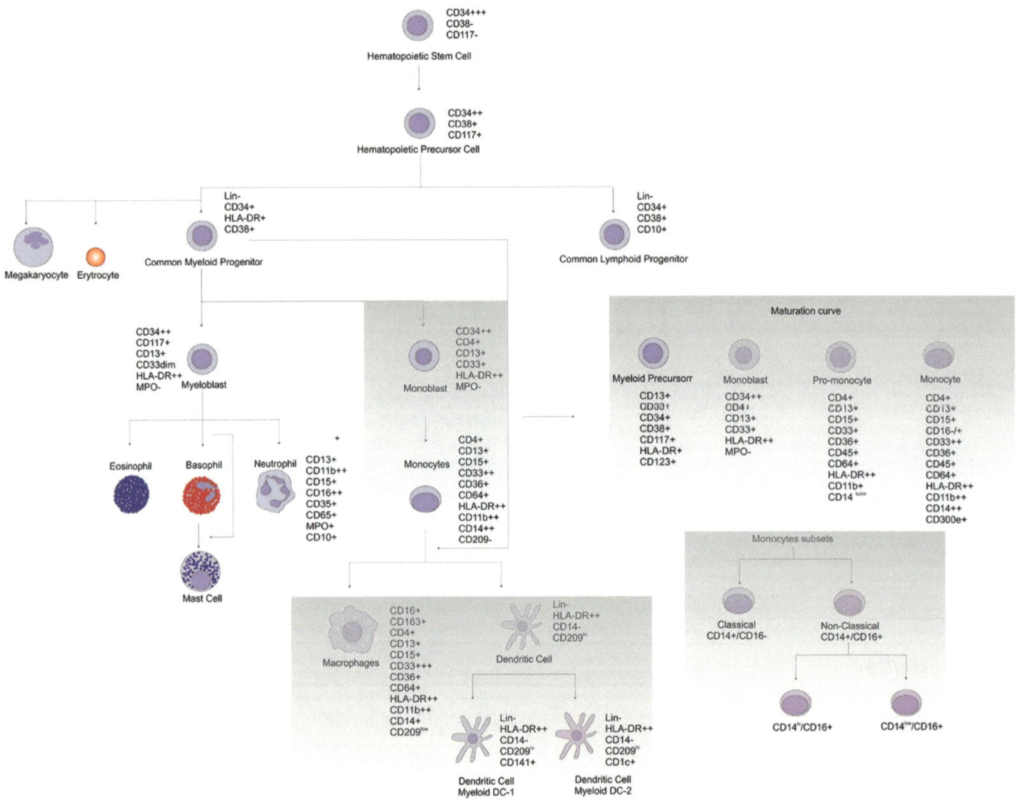

Figure 1. Hematopoiesis—General representation of hematopoiesis with focus on myelomonocitic differentiation [1, 2].

Myeloid cells represent the major leukocyte population in the peripheral blood. Phylogenically, these cells are the oldest ones found in primitive invertebrates and, in vertebrates, sum to lymphoid cells to constantly supply to all tissues via peripheral blood circulation [1].

The myeloid precursor gives rise to granulocytes and monocytes. Granulocytes are comprised of neutrophils, eosinophils, and basophils. Neutrophils are known as the key effector cells in innate immunity against bacteria and are the first cells to be recruited into local sites on pathogen invasion, providing an immediate defense against infection in tissues. The main role of neutrophils is to isolate, engulf, and kill pathogens using oxidative and nonoxidative mechanisms [1, 2].

Myelomonocytic cells give rise to mature monocytes that are present in circulation and were believed to mature terminally into macrophages in various tissues, where they may display a unique, tissue-dependent morphology and specific functions such as Kupffer cells in the liver or microglia in the brain. Monocytes may also differentiate into dendritic cells in lymphoid organs and Langerhans cells in skin, where they function as professional antigen presenting cells [2].

Monocytes, dendritic cells, and macrophages are the bridge between innate and adaptive immunity, they are a group of cells that are vital for the control of pathogens and for orchestration of a complete immune response, as well as for backing up tissue functions. These

http://dx.doi.org/10.5772/67324

properties make them interesting targets for immune therapy, vaccination, and treatment of autoimmune and inflammatory diseases [3, 4].

However, exactly how many cell types exist in the mononuclear phagocyte system, or whether they establish a family, has been a matter of discussion for many years. Historically, cells of the mononuclear phagocyte system have been referred to as erythrophagocytes, adventitia cells, histiocytes, and several other terminologies until their current terminology was established in 1972 by a bulletin published by the World Health Organization (WHO) [5]. The discovery of a new cell type termed dendritic cells in the 1970s by the Nobel Prize winner Ralph Steinman that was distinct from macrophages added more complexity to the mononuclear phagocyte system classification [6].

Accordingly, it took a while before dendritic cells were fully accepted as a true member of the mononuclear phagocyte system. Over time, there was appreciation that there were not just one but multiple dendritic cells subtypes, each with a specialized role [7]. Nowadays, there are several discussions about macrophages and dendritic cells nomenclature, subsets, and their *in vivo* origin, and how much they are related to macrophages or monocytes.

Thus in this chapter, the principles of hematopoiesis, phenotype, and transcription factors in myelomonocytic lineage will be highlighted, as well as their maturation and differentiation. The contribution of different cytokine environments modulating the monocytic lineage differentiation into subtypes of macrophages or dendritic cells will also be discussed.

2. Hematopoiesis, phenotype, and lineage transcription factors

Blood development in vertebrates includes two hematopoiesis waves: primitive and definitive ones [8]. The primitive wave involves an erythroid progenitor and gives rise to erythrocytes and macrophages during the early embryonic development [9]. The purpose of the primitive wave is to produce red blood cells in order to oxygenate the embryo tissues that experience a fast growth [10]. In mammals, these erythroid progenitor cells first appear in blood islands in the extra-embryonic yolk sac early in development [11]. The primitive wave is transitory, and these erythroid progenitors are not pluripotent and do not have self-renewal ability.

Instead, definitive hematopoiesis occurs later in development, markedly at different periods in different species. Definitive hematopoiesis involves hematopoietic stem cells, which are multipotent cells that can generate all blood lineages of an adult organism. In vertebrates, hematopoietic stem cells are born in the aorta-gonad-mesonephros region of the developing embryo. They migrate to the fetal liver and then to the bone marrow, which is the final site for hematopoietic stem cells in adults [12].

Usually, in order to characterize and quantify hematopoietic stem cells, flow cytometry techniques are commonly used. The immunophenotypic markers CD34 and CD38 are used to characterize and enumerate hematopoietic stem cell (HSC) and progenitors (HPC) as shown in **Figures 1** and **2** [13]. Hematopoietic stem cells are a small population characterized by the expression of CD34+CD38−, and progenitors are recognized by the expression of CD34+CD38+

(**Figure 2A**). HSCs are also CD117−, and during differentiation toward common myeloid and lymphoid progenitors (CMP and CLP), they acquire CD117 and Human Leukocyte Antigen–DR (HLA-DR) expression; and later, as per their lineage commitment, they can or not preserve these markers (**Figure 2B**).

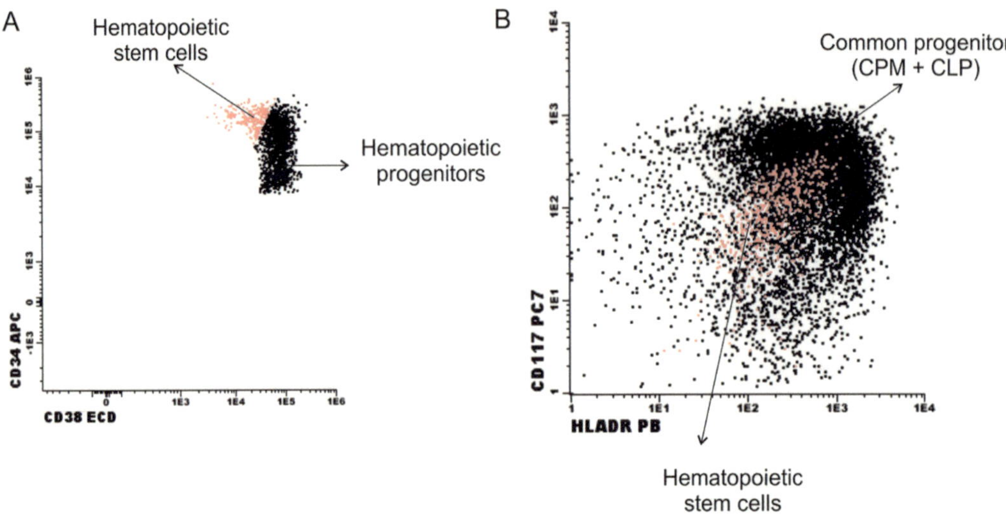

Figure 2. Hematopoietic stem cells differentiation curve—(A) Hematopoietic progenitors CD34+CD38+, hematopoietic stem cells CD34+CD38− (red). **(B)** Common myeloid and lymphoid progenitors (CMP and CLP) are CD34+CD38+CD117+HLA-DR+ (black) (Infinicyt software was used for this analysis, Cytognos).

After hematopoiesis initiation, several decision steps are necessary for HSC pluripotency and quiescence maintenance or specification of lineage commitment [14]. One important checkpoint is the preservation of pluripotency by the combined action of Notch-1, GATA-2, HoxB4, and Ikaros transcription factors. Furthermore, the cell cycle inhibitor p21 is essential to keep a fraction of stem cells in quiescence [15].

During lineage commitment, transcription factors play critical roles at distinct differentiation branches. Concerning the myeloid-lineage commitment, PU.1, an Ets family of transcription factor, seems to play a key role [16]. PU.1-deficient mice lack monocytes and B cells with a greatly reduced number of granulocytes, while overexpression of PU.1 enhances the development of myeloid cells. Consequently, the enhanced expression of PU.1 favors myeloid commitment, while low-to-intermediate expression of PU.1 together with GATA-3 and Ikaros transcription factors commit HSC toward lymphoid lineage [17].

Once the myeloid dominance has been established through increased PU.1 or GATA-1 expression, further transcriptional control determines the commitment along erythroid/megakaryocytic (GATA-1/2 dominance) or myelomonocytic (PU.1 dominance) lineages, while mafB together with PU.1 also play an essential role in monocyte/macrophage differentiation [18]. MafB, c-Maf, and Egr-1 are suggested to promote monocytic differentiation at the cost of granulopoiesis [19].

In addition, the induction of C/EBPα or C/EBPβ modulates the fate of myeloid-committed cells toward granulocytic branches since CCAAT/Enhancer Binding Protein (C/EBP), a basic region leucine zipper DNA-binding protein, is responsible for the transactivation of Granulocyte-Colony Stimulating Factor Receptor (G-CSFR) gene and retinoic acid receptors (RARs) [14]. It has been shown that C/EBP-deficient mice selectively lacks granulocytes and RAR-deficient mice shows a granulocyte differentiation arrested at the myelocyte stage.

Myelomonocytic cells are usually classified based on surface markers and biological responses. The common myeloid progenitor (CMP) is characterized by markers such as CD34 and CD117. These immature cells are able to differentiate into neutrophils, monocytes, macrophages, dendritic cells (DCs), and under pathological conditions or induced by proinflammatory cytokines these cells can also generate a population known as myeloid-derived suppressor cells.

Myeloid-derived suppressor cells are part of the myeloid-cell lineage and a heterogeneous population that is comprised by myeloid-progenitors and precursors cells. In healthy individuals, immature myeloid cells rapidly differentiate toward mature granulocytes, macrophages, or dendritic cells. However, in pathological conditions such as cancer, infectious diseases, trauma, or some autoimmune disorders, a partial impairment in the immature myeloid cells differentiation result in the expansion of this population. Importantly, the activation of these cells in pathological conditions results in an upregulated expression of immune suppressive factors such as arginase, inducible nitric oxide synthase (iNOS), and reactive oxygen species (ROS) increased production. Together, these alterations results in the expansion of immature myeloid cells that possess suppressive activity [20].

3. Monocytes maturation curve and subsets

Regarding phenotypes, monocyte maturation curve can be performed by flow cytometry and can display the differentiation of CD34+/CD117+/CD64−/CD14− myeloid precursor into monoblast CD64+ and further into promonocyte by increased expression of $CD14^{lo/int}$. Additionally, these cells will become full mature monocytes by $CD14^{hi}$ expression (**Figures 1** and **3A**). During monocyte maturation, upregulation of CD64 is followed not only by CD14 but also increased levels of CD33, CD36, and CD300e expression toward mature monocytes (**Figures 1** and **3A**).

In addition, the differences in monocytes and granulocytes maturation curve can be seen using a combination of CD11b and HLA-DR markers. Granulocytes arise from a precursor that do express HLA-DR and downregulated its expression during maturation, while monocytes arise from a precursor with high expression of HLA-DR and preserve the HLA-DR expression to maturation, while both cells' subsets have an increased expression of CD11b toward maturation (**Figures 1** and **3B**).

Monocytes were originally classified by their physical characteristics, but after flow cytometry advent, monocytes became also recognized by CD14 and CD16 expressions (**Figures 1** and **4A**). Classical monocytes $CD14^{hi}$/CD16− (**Figures 1** and **4B**) are approximately 80% of all monocytes and considered to be better at secreting proinflammatory cytokines, phagocytosis, and ROS production [21]. The nonclassical CD14+/CD16+ cells resemble "resident" tissue macrophages with higher Major Histocompatibility Complex - Class II (MHC-II) expression. CD16+ monocytes

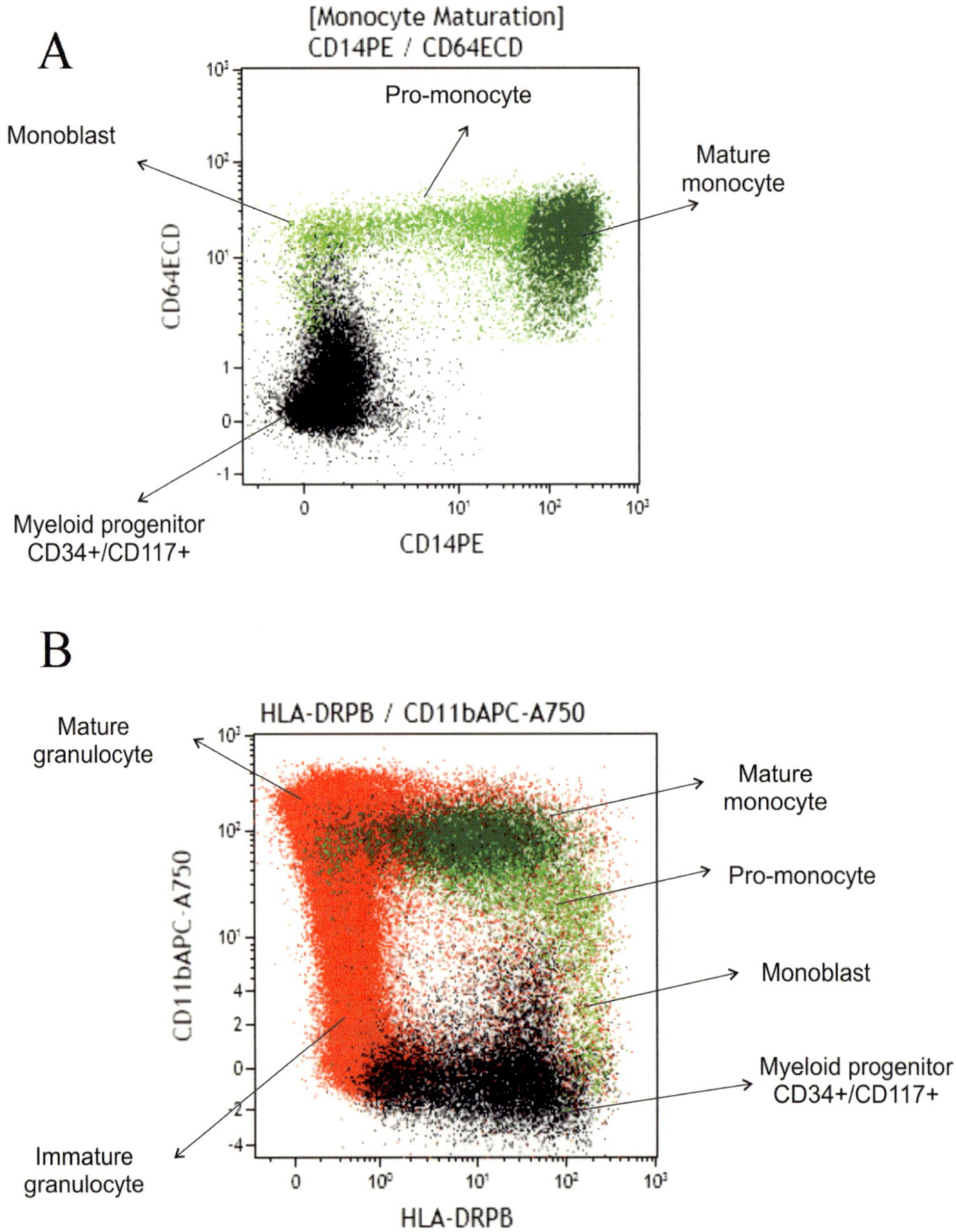

Figure 3. Monocyte and granulocyte maturation curve—(A) Monocyte maturation: this dot plot displays a combination of previously three-gated population and shows myeloid progenitors CD34+/CD117+/CD64−/CD14− (black), monoblast CD64+CD14− and promonocytes CD64+CD14$^{lo/int}$ (light green), mature monocyte CD64+CD14^{hi} (dark green). **(B) Monocyte and granulocyte maturation**: this dot plot displays a combination of previously four-gated population and shows myeloid progenitors CD34+/CD117+/HLA-DR+ (black), monoblast HLADR+CD14− and promonocytes HLA-DR$^{lo/int}$ (light green), mature monocyte HLA-DR+CD14^{hi} (dark green), immature granulocytes HLA-DR−/CD11b^{lo}, and mature granulocytes HLA-DR−/CD11b^{hi} (red) (Kalusa software was used for this analysis, Beckman Coulter).

are subdivided into CD14^{hi}/CD16+ and CD14^{lo}/CD16+ (**Figures 1** and **4B**). CD14^{hi}/CD16+ monocytes express highest levels of phagocytosis; MHC-II and accessory molecule expression are also higher compared with CD14^{lo}/CD16+ (**Figures 1** and **4C**) [21]. Functional data and gene arrays suggest that CD14^{hi}/CD16+ monocytes share more common pattern with CD14^{hi}/CD16− monocytes than with CD14^{lo}/CD16+ [22].

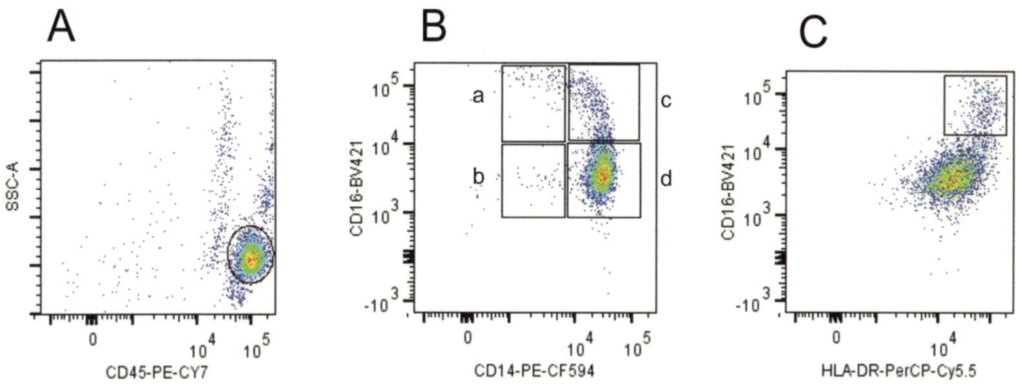

Figure 4. Monocytes (CD14+) sorted from human peripheral blood—(A) SSC vs CD45. **(B)** Monocytes subpopulations (a) CD14^{lo}/CD16+ (b) CD14^{lo}/CD16− (c) CD14^{hi}/CD16+ and (d) CD14^{hi}/CD16−. **(C)** CD14^{hi} (c+d)/CD16+ are HLA-DR^{hi} (FlowJo software was used for this analysis, TreeStar).

These monocyte characteristics subsets have recently been reported as a signature diagnostic for chronic myelomonocytic leukemia (CMML). Researchers compared the population of monocytes among healthy bone marrow donors, patients with reactive monocytosis, another hematologic malignancy, and CMML patients, which demonstrate a characteristic increase in the fraction of CD14+/CD16− cells compared with the other samples [23].

In addition, the development and biological significance of monocyte subsets remain a matter of active investigation, as well as their respective functions and developmental relationships. CD161 is another important marker that also defines monocytes subsets. These CD161 subsets seem to be expanded in a variety of clinical situations, including autoimmune diseases, bacterial and viral infections, asthma, stroke, and coronary artery disease [24–29]. In addition, there is a new emerging technology known as tissue macrophage scanning (TiMaScan), which is a sensitive intra-tissue total body scanning. This new technology promises to accurately detect and define monocyte and macrophage subsets in blood and tissues not only in homeostatic or traumatic injuries but also in cancer [30, 31].

Monocytes, macrophages, and myeloid DCs are members of the mononuclear phagocyte system that exhibit several functions during immune responses. Historically, these cells have been grouped together because although monocytes have their unique functions as mononuclear phagocytic cells, they were also considered as precursors of macrophages and myeloid DCs [32].

Monocytes and macrophages are critical effectors and regulators of inflammation involved in innate immune response, the immune system for immediate support. On the other hand, DCs are a bridge between innate and adaptive immunity, because they initiate and regulate the highly pathogen-specific adaptive immune responses and play a central role in the development of immunological memory and tolerance. These cells can display significant heterogeneity in phenotype and function according to the tissue of residence. Dendritic cells are described as distinct lineage specialized in antigen presentation, initiation, and control of immunity, contributing to development of the immune response to pathogens, vaccines, and tumors [33].

Human dendritic cells subsets found *in vivo* are described in the literature as two main groups, plasmacytoid DCs (pDCs) and *classical* or *myeloid* DCs. Classical or myeloid DCs have been further subdivided into two subsets on the basis of their CD141 expression (also known as BDCA3) and CD1c (also known as BDCA1) [34, 35]. It has been shown that the gene-expression profiles and functions of human CD141+ DCs and CD1c+ DCs resemble those of mouse cDC1s and cDC2s, respectively [36].

Regarding transcription factors that regulate monocytes and DCs differentiation, there are several differences between mice and humans, but also similarities, which should be taken into consideration [37]. A straight comparison between human and mouse can be made due to the presence of Interferon Regulatory Factor 8 (IRF8) deficiency in both species. While human biallelic IRF8 mutation leads to complete loss of blood and skin DCs and monocytes derived cells, the autosomal dominant IRF8 mutation results in absence of CD1c expression and presence of a population CD11c+CD1c− not seen in a healthy control blood [37, 38]. In mice, IRF8 is required for the development of CD8+CD103+ DCs and plays a role in monocyte development through Interferon Regulatory Factor (IRF) interaction with Krüppel-like Factor 4 (KLF4) [39].

In contrast, human macrophages are found throughout body tissues [40]. During HSC transplantation, dermal macrophages in the recipient show prolonged survival and delayed replacement compared with dermal DCs, which is consistent with the impression that macrophages are also self-maintaining in humans. Furthermore, patients carrying a mutation in GATA-2 lack blood monocytes and all conventional DCs subsets, yet they have normal numbers of Langerhans cells and macrophages in skin and lungs, respectively, suggesting that these populations development may also occur independent of monocytes and DCs [41].

Another important characteristic of macrophages, which should be mentioned, is their polarization in two phenotypes M1 and M2, inflammatory macrophages are called M1, whereas those that decrease inflammation and favor tissue repair are called M2 macrophages. Later, findings regarding granulocyte macrophage colony-stimulating factor (GM-CSF) and macrophage colony-stimulating factor (M-CSF) effects in macrophages led to the independent inclusion of these as M1 and M2 stimuli, respectively. The polarized M2 phenotype, in a tumor microenvironment, has been named tumor-associated macrophages (TAMs) and is associated to tumor progression and to a poor prognosis [42].

4. Cytokines, growth factors, and *in vitro* models of monocyte differentiation into dendritic cells and macrophages

It is possible to differentiate either dendritic cells or macrophages *in vitro* from monocytes using differential growth factors, and these cells are differentiated from those found *in vivo* by being named as monocyte-derived cells. A number of growth factors have been shown to influence monocyte development and differentiation into macrophages, and the best-recognized growth factor is the macrophage colony-stimulating factor (M-CSF). Its significance involves the observation that circulating monocytes express the M-CSF receptor [43, 44] and administration of M-CSF drives monocytosis [45–47].

Moreover, mice deficient either in the production of Macrophage-Colony Stimulating Factor (M-CSF) or in the Macrophage-Colony Stimulating Factor Receptor (M-CSFR) have been reported to have decreased numbers of monocytes in the bone marrow and/or in circulation [48]. Homeostatic control of monocyte/macrophage development has been proposed to result from the modulation of M-CSF levels by differentiated cells of the mononuclear phagocyte system, mature mononuclear phagocytes express high levels of the M-CSFR, and M-CSF is produced continuously by stromal cells, and the addition of IL-3 to cultured bone marrow cells enhances the activity of M-CSF [49].

Additional growth factors, including granulocyte-macrophage colony-stimulating factor (GM-CSF) and IL-4, are able to influence monocyte development and differentiation during inflammation. *In vitro* GM-CSF supports monocyte expansion and differentiation [50, 51]. Unexpectedly, GM-CSF deficient mice show minimal perturbation of hematopoiesis and no decrease in circulating monocyte numbers compared with the control [52]. However, *in vivo*, GM-CSF is not produced at high levels under homeostatic conditions; instead, it is upregulated during inflammation [50, 51]. This suggests that, in contrast to M-CSF, GM-CSF primarily contributes to monopoiesis during inflammatory states. Accordingly, M-CSF and GM-CSF drive different differentiation platforms, with M-CSF stimulation leading to a homeostatic phenotype, and GM-CSF stimulation leading to monocytes with an inflammatory phenotype. In addition, GM-CSF was the first growth factor shown to efficiently promote dendritic cells development *in vitro* and has been used to induce dendritic cell differentiation from human monocytes, as well as human and mouse hematopoietic progenitor cells [53, 54].

IL-4 has been argued to drive both tissue-resident macrophage [55, 56] and monocyte [57] expansion during type 2 inflammation. IL-4 in combination with GM-CSF drives inflammatory dendritic cells *in vitro* [53]. Studies in both Signal Transducer and Activator of Transcription 6 (STAT6) [57] and IL-4R [55] deficient mice indicate that IL-4-dependent signaling does not contribute to monocyte development during homeostasis.

The two main colony-stimulating factors involved in monopoiesis, M-CSF and GM-CSF, have opposing polarizing properties. *In vitro*, M-CSF supports the development of cells with anti-inflammatory profile that is characterized by production of IL-10 and CCL2 but not IL-12 or IL-23 [58]. On the other hand, culture of either bone marrow or purified monocytes with GM-CSF leads to upregulation of MHC class II as well as induction of IL-12 and IL-23, but minimal IL-10 production [59]. Based on these data, it has been discussed that M-CSF stimulation represents a homeostatic/M2 pathway for monocyte development [60]. *In vivo*, GM-CSF has been shown to induce an inflammatory DC/M1-like phenotype in monocytes in a variety of models [61].

Macrophages *in vitro* monocyte-derived, using M-CSF, are distinguished as larger and vacuolar cells, been very effective at apoptotic cells, cellular debris and pathogens clearance, and can be differentiated from DCs, monocytes-derived with GM-CSF in combination with IL-4 *in vitro* by the CD14 expression and from monocytes by CD209 (DC-SIGN) expression. By contrast, DCs are defined with stellate morphology that can efficiently present antigens

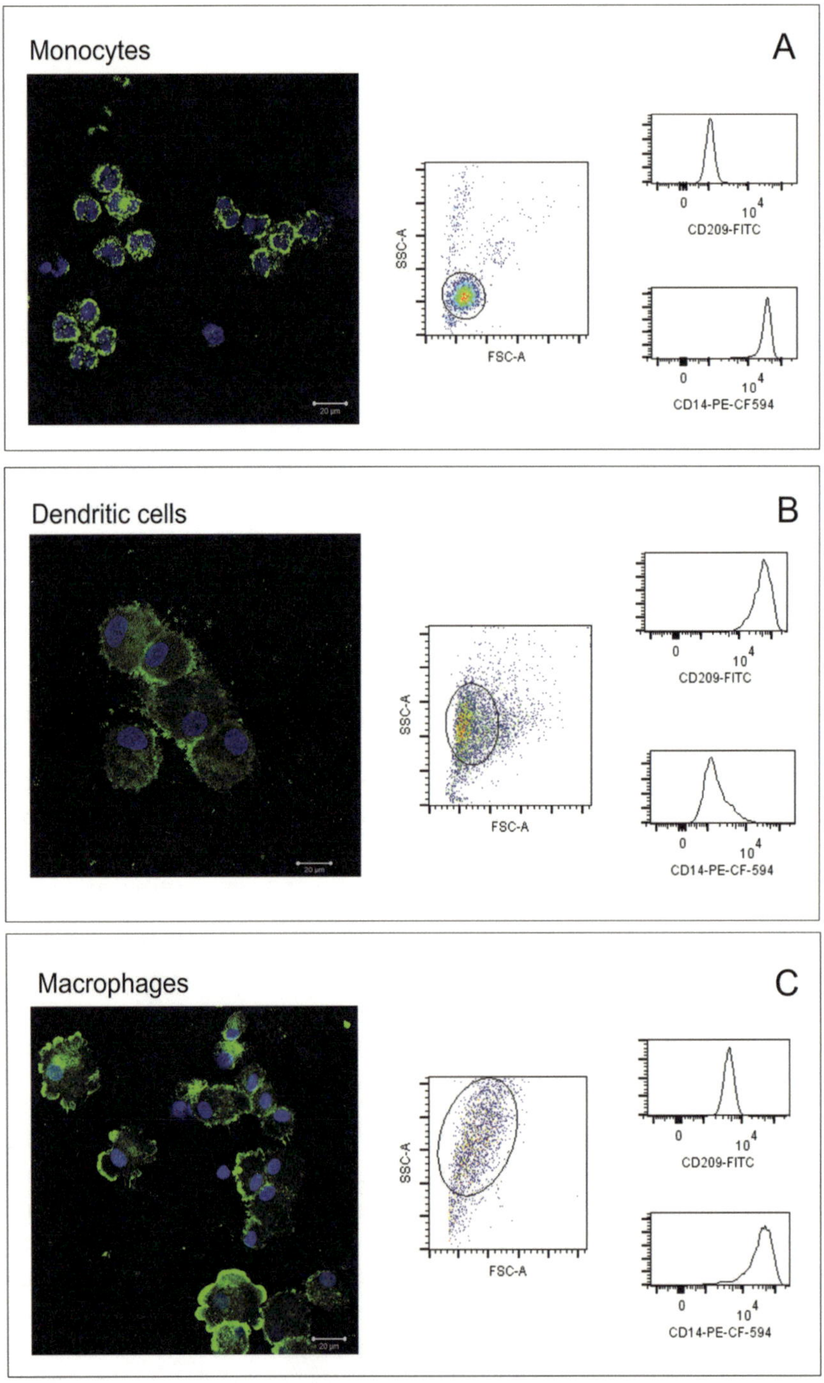

Figure 5. Monocytes, dendritic cells, and macrophages morphology and phenotype—To confocal microscopy analysis, all cells were stained with pan-actin (green) in order to show differences in morphology and cytoskeleton, and the nucleus were stained with DAPI (blue): (A) monocytes CD14+/CD209–, (B) dendritic cells CD14–/CD209^{hi}, (C) macrophages CD14+/CD209^{int} (FlowJo software was used for this analysis, TreeStar).

through MHC molecules and activate naïve T cells. DCs derived from monocytes lack CD14 and acquire CD209 expression (**Figures 1** and **5**).

Regarding phagocytosis, monocytes and macrophages are highly phagocytic cells, in contrast to DCs that according to maturation status lose their phagocytic ability and become the most efficient antigen-presenting cells. Differences in expression related to functional status

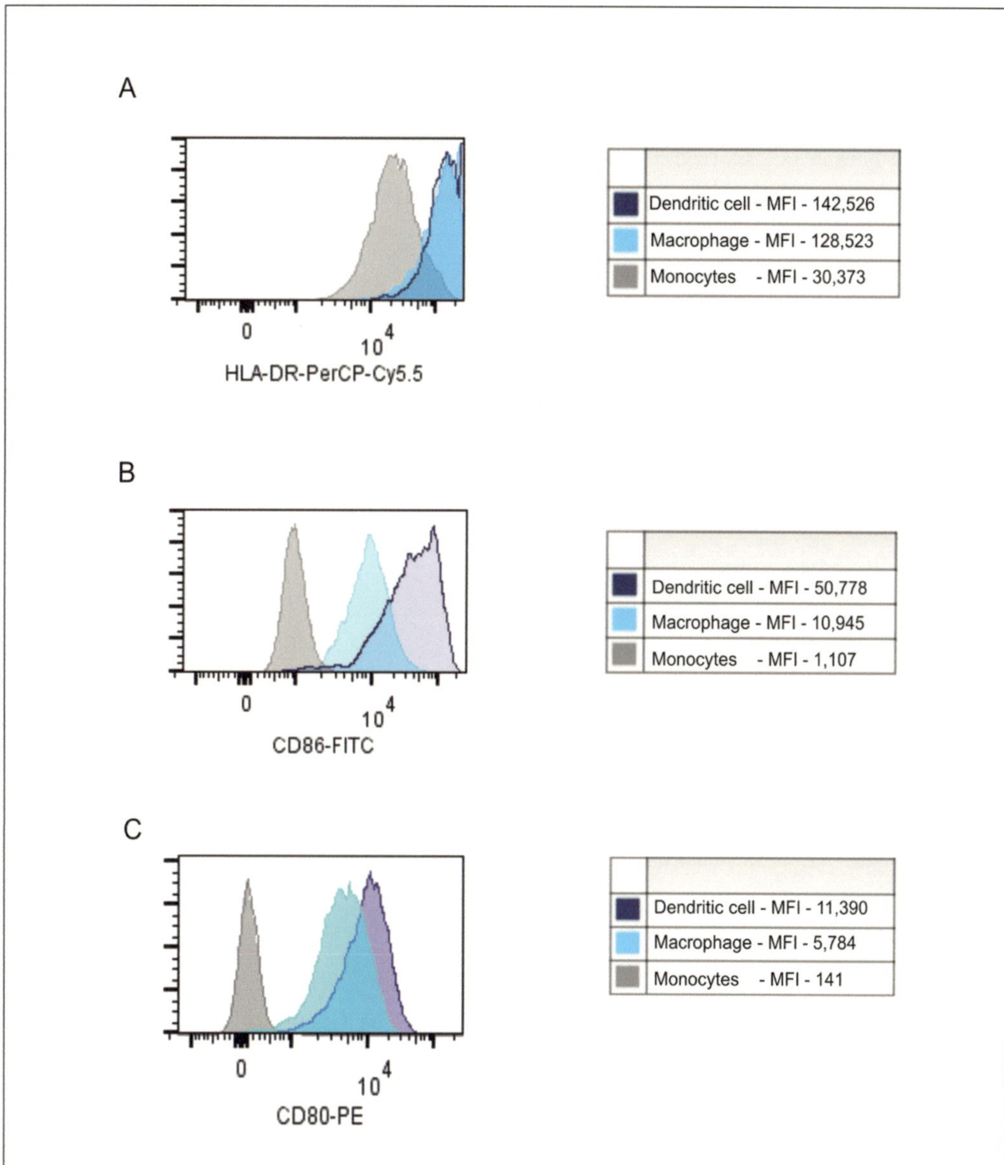

Figure 6. Monocytes, dendritic cells, and macrophages expression of HLA-DR, CD80, and CD86—(A) HLA-DR, (B) CD86, (C) CD80 increasing expression in media fluorescence intensity (MFI) (FlowJo software was used for this analysis, TreeStar).

of these cells are shown in **Figures 5** and **6**. DCs have increased expression in HLA-DR, CD80 and CD86 (molecules related to antigen presentation efficiency) compared with macrophages and monocytes (**Figure 6**).

5. Concluding remarks

Herein, we have presented the principles of hematopoiesis, transcription factors in myelomonocytic lineage phenotype, as well as their maturation and differentiation, and these topics have been the target of several studies for over a century using a variety of model systems. The human hematopoiesis understanding it is very important; this fundamental knowledge allowed scientists and physicians to identify diseases and their causes, leading to the development of new therapies.

In addition, we have discussed the contribution of different cytokine/growth factors' environment, modulating the monocytic lineage differentiation into subtypes of macrophages or dendritic cells and their development *in vitro*. Similarities and differences between cells found *in vivo* with the ones generated *in vitro* are very important for the development of new study models. Furthermore, the comprehension about growth factors and how to use them to modulate cells can favor their application in developmental hematology and immunology. These topics are very important for the continuous development of knowledge.

Acknowledgements

This work was granted by National Counsel of Technological and Scientific Development (CNPq) process number—441665/2014-4. We are grateful to Dr. Thiago Aloia by performing the confocal microscopy images and to Sociedade Beneficente Israelita Brasileira Hospital Albert Einstein and Clinical Pathology Laboratory for all support.

Author details

Luciana Cavalheiro Marti[1]*, Nydia Strachman Bacal[2], Laiz Camerão Bento[2] and Fernanda Agostini Rocha[2]

*Address all correspondence to: luciana.marti@einstein.br

1 Experimental Research Center, Hospital Israelita Albert Einstein, São Paulo, Brazil

2 Hospital Israelita Albert Einstein, São Paulo, Brazil

References

[1] Kawamoto H and Minato N. Myeloid cells. Int J Biochem Cell Biol. 2004; 36(8):1374–9.

[2] Hickey MJ and Kubes P. Intravascular immunity: the host-pathogen encounter in blood vessels. Nat Rev Immunol. 2009; 9(5):364–75.

[3] Ginhoux F and Jung S. Monocytes and macrophages: developmental pathways and tissue homeostasis. Nat Rev Immunol. 2014; 14:392–404.

[4] Schlitzer A and Ginhoux F. Organization of the mouse and human DC network. Curr Opin Immunol. 2014; 26:90–9.

[5] van Furth R, Cohn ZA, Hirsch JG, Humphrey JH, Spector WG and Langevoort HL. The mononuclear phagocyte system: a new classification of macrophages, monocytes, and their precursor cells. Bull World Health Organ. 1972; 46:845–52.

[6] Steinman RM and Cohn ZA. Identification of a novel cell type in peripheral lymphoid organs of mice. I. Morphology, quantitation, tissue distribution. J Exp Med. 1973; 137:1142–62.

[7] Schlitzer A, McGovern N and Ginhoux F. Dendritic cells and monocyte-derived cells: two complementary and integrated functional systems. Semin Cell Dev Biol. 2015; 41:9–22.

[8] Galloway J and Land Zon LI. Ontogeny of hematopoiesis: examining the emergence of hematopoietic cells in the vertebrate embryo. Curr Top Dev Biol. 2003; 53:139–58.

[9] Palis J and Yoder MC. Yolk-sac hematopoiesis: the first blood cells of mouse and man. Exp Hematol. 2001; 29:927–36.

[10] Orkin SH and Zon LI. Hematopoiesis: an evolving paradigm for stem cell biology. Cell. 2008; 132:631–44.

[11] Paik EJ and Zon LI. Hematopoietic development in the zebrafish. Int J Dev Biol. 2010; 54:1127–37.

[12] Cumano A and Godin I. Ontogeny of the hematopoietic system. Annu Rev Immunol. 2007; 25:745–85.

[13] Terstappen LW, Huang S, Safford M, Lansdorp PM and Loken MR. Sequential generations of hematopoietic colonies derived from single nonlineage-committed $CD34^{+}CD38^{-}$ progenitor cells. Blood. 1991; 77:1218–27.

[14] Aggarwal R, Lu J, Pompili VJ and Das H. Hematopoietic stem cells: transcriptional regulation, ex vivo expansion and clinical application. Curr Mol Med. 2012; 12(1):34–49.

[15] Cheng T, Rodrigues N, Shen H, Yang Y, Dombkowski D, Sykes M and Scadden DT. Hematopoietic stem cell quiescence maintained by p21cip1/waf1. Science. 2000; 287(5459):1804–8.

[16] DeKoter RP and Singh H. Regulation of B lymphocyte and macrophage development by graded expression of PU.1. Science. 2000; 288:1439–41.

[17] Orkin SH. Diversification of haematopoietic stem cells to specific lineages. Nat Rev Genet. 2000; 1(1):57–64.

[18] Kelly LM, Englmeier U, Lafon I, Sieweke MH and Graf T. MafB is an inducer of monocytic differentiation. EMBO J. 2000; 19(9):1987–97.

[19] Friedman AD. Transcriptional regulation of granulocyte and monocyte development. Oncogene. 2002; 21:3377–90.

[20] Gabrilovich DI and Nagaraj S. Myeloid-derived suppressor cells as regulators of the immune system. Nat Rev Immunol. 2009; 9(3):162–74.

[21] Abeles RD, McPhail MJ, Sowter D, Antoniades CG, Vergis N, Vijay GK, Xystrakis E, Khamri W, Shawcross DL, Ma Y, Wendon JA and Vergani D. CD14, CD16 and HLA-DR reliably identifies human monocytes and their subsets in the context of pathologically reduced HLA-DR expression by CD14(hi)/CD16(neg) monocytes: expansion of CD14(hi)/CD16(pos) and contraction of CD14(lo)/CD16(pos) monocytes in acute liver failure. Cytometry A. 2012; 81(10):823–34.

[22] Cros J, Cagnard N, Woollard K, Patey N, Zhang SY, Senechal B, Puel A, Biswas SK, Moshous D, Picard C, Jais JP, D'Cruz D, Casanova JL, Trouillet C and Geissmann F. Human CD14dim monocytes patrol and sense nucleic acids and viruses via TLR7 and TLR8 receptors. Immunity. 2010; 33(3):375–86.

[23] Selimoglu-Buet D, Wagner-Ballon O, Saada V, Bardet V, Itzykson R, Morabito LBM, Met E, Debord C, Benayoun E, Nloga AM, Fenaux P, Braun T, Willekens C, Quesnel B, Adès L, Fontenay M, Rameau P, Droin N, Koscielny S and Solary E. Characteristic repartition of monocyte subsets as a diagnostic signature of chronic myelomonocytic leukemia. Blood. 2015; 125:3618–26.

[24] Auffray C, Sieweke MH and Geissmann F. Blood monocytes: development, heterogeneity, and relationship with dendritic cells. Annu Rev Immunol. 2009; 27:669–92.

[25] Rogacev KS, Cremers B, Zawada AM, Seiler S, Binder N, Ege P, Große-Dunker G, Heisel I, Hornof F, Jeken J, Rebling NM, Ulrich C, Scheller B, Böhm M, Fliser D and Heine GH. CD1411CD161 monocytes independently predict cardiovascular events: a cohort study of 951 patients referred for elective coronary angiography. J Am Coll Cardiol. 2012; 60(16):1512–20.

[26] Hanna RN, Shaked I, Hubbeling HG, Punt JA, Wu R, Herrley E, Zaugg C, Pei H, Geissmann F, Ley K and Hedrick CC. NR4A1 (Nur77) deletion polarizes macrophages toward an inflammatory phenotype and increases atherosclerosis. Circ Res. 2012; 110(3):416–27.

[27] Rossol M, Kraus S, Pierer M, Baerwald C and Wagner U. The CD14(bright) CD161 monocyte subset is expanded in rheumatoid arthritis and promotes expansion of the Th17 cell population. Arthritis Rheum. 2012; 64(3):671–7.

[28] Fingerle G, Pforte A, Passlick B, Blumenstein M, Ströbel M and Ziegler-Heitbrock HW. The novel subset of CD141/CD161 blood monocytes is expanded in sepsis patients. Blood. 1993; 82(10):3170–6.

[29] Skrzeczyñska J, Kobylarz K, Hartwich Z, Zembala M, Pryjma J. CD141CD161 monocytes in the course of sepsis in neonates and small children: monitoring and functional studies. Scand J Immunol. 2002; 55(6):629–38.

[30] Van Dongen JJ and Orfao A. Methods and means for monitoring disruption of tissue homeostasis in the total body. EP 12709398.7 (Patent) 2011.

[31] Damasceno D, Andrés MP, van den Bossche WB, Flores-Montero J, de Bruin S, Teodosio C, van Dongen JJ, Orfao A, Almeida J. Expression profile of novel cell surface molecules on different subsets of human peripheral blood antigen-presenting cells. Clin Transl Immunology. 2016 Sep 16;5(9):e100.

[32] Chomarat P, Banchereau J, Davoust J and Palucka AK. IL-6 switches the differentiation of monocytes from dendritic cells to macrophages. Nat Immunol. 2000; 1(6):510–4.

[33] Steinman RM, Lustig DS, Cohn ZA. Identification of a novel cell type in peripheral lymphoid organs of mice. 3. Functional properties in vivo. J Exp Med. 1974 Jun 1;139(6):1431–45.

[34] Haniffa M, Shin A, Bigley V, McGovern N, Teo P, See P, Wasan PS, Wang XN, Malinarich F, Malleret B, Larbi A, Tan P, Zhao H, Poidinger M, Pagan S, Cookson S, Dickinson R, Dimmick I, Jarrett RF, Renia L, Tam J, Song C, Connolly J, Chan JK, Gehring A, Bertoletti A, Collin M and Ginhoux F. Human tissues contain CD141hi cross-presenting dendritic cells with functional homology to mouse CD103+ nonlymphoid dendritic cells. Immunity. 2013; 37:60–73.

[35] Yu CI, Becker C, Wang Y, Marches F, Helft J, Leboeuf M, Anguiano E, Pourpe S, Goller K, Pascual V, Banchereau J, Merad M and Palucka K. Human CD1c+ dendritic cells drive the differentiation of CD103+ CD8+ mucosal effector T cells via the cytokine TGF-β. Immunity. 2013; 38:818–30.

[36] Jongbloed SL, Kassianos AJ, McDonald KJ, Clark GJ, Ju X, Angel CE, Chen CJ, Dunbar PR, Wadley RB, Jeet V, Vulink AJ, Hart DN and Radford KJ. Human CD141+ (BDCA-3)+ dendritic cells (DCs) represent a unique myeloid DC subset that cross-presents necrotic cell antigens. J Exp Med. 2010; 207:1247–60.

[37] Haniffa M, Bigley V and Collin M. Human mononuclear phagocyte system reunited. Semin Cell Dev Biol. 2015; 41:59–69.

[38] Hambleton S, Salem S, Bustamante J, Bigley V, Boisson-Dupuis S, Azevedo J, Fortin A, Haniffa M, Ceron-Gutierrez L, Bacon CM, Menon G, Trouillet C, McDonald D, Carey

P, Ginhoux F, Alsina L, Zumwalt TJ, Kong XF, Kumararatne D, Butler K, Hubeau M, Feinberg J, Al-Muhsen S, Cant A, Abel L, Chaussabel D, Doffinger R, Talesnik E, Grumach A, Duarte A, Abarca K, Moraes-Vasconcelos D, Burk D, Berghuis A, Geissmann F, Collin M, Casanova JL and Gros P. IRF8 mutations and human dendritic-cell immunodeficiency. N Engl J Med. 2011; 365:127–38.

[39] Kurotaki D, Osato N, Nishiyama A, Yamamoto M, Ban T, Sato H, Nakabayashi J, Umehara M, Miyake N, Matsumoto N, Nakazawa M, Ozato K and Tamura T. Essential role of the IRF8-KLF4 transcription factor cascade in murine monocyte differentiation. Blood. 2013; 121:1839–49.

[40] Guilliams M, Ginhoux F, Jakubzick C, Naik SH, Onai N, Schraml BU, Segura E, Tussiwand R and Yona S. Dendritic cells, monocytes and macrophages: a unified nomenclature based on ontogeny. Nat Rev Immunol. 2014; 14(8):571–8.

[41] Watchmaker PB, Lahl K, Lee M, Baumjohann D, Morton J, Kim SJ, Zeng R, Dent A, Ansel KM, Diamond B, Hadeiba H and Butcher EC. Comparative transcriptional and functional profiling defines conserved programs of intestinal DC differentiation in humans and mice. Nat Immunol. 2014; 15(1):98–108.

[42] Rhee I. Diverse macrophages polarization in tumor microenvironment. Arch Pharm Res. 2016; 39(11):1588–96.

[43] Sunderkotter C, Nikolic T, Dillon MJ, Van RN, Stehling M, Drevets DA and Leenen PJ. Subpopulations of mouse blood monocytes differ in maturation stage and inflammatory response. J Immunol. 2004; 172:4410–7.

[44] Ingersoll MA, Spanbroek R, Lottaz C, Gautier EL, Frankenberger M, Hoffmann R, Lang R, Haniffa M, Collin M, Tacke F, Habenicht AJR, Ziegler-Heitbrock L and Randolph GJ. Comparison of gene expression profiles between human and mouse monocyte subsets. Blood. 2010; 115:e10–9.

[45] Hume DA, Pavli P, Donahue RE and Fidler IJ. The effect of human recombinant macrophage colony-stimulating factor (CSF-1) on the murine mononuclear phagocyte system in vivo. J Immunol. 1998; 141:3405–9.

[46] Weiner LM, Li W, Holmes M, Catalano RB, Dovnarsky M, Padavic K and Alpaugh RK. Phase I trial of recombinant macrophage colony-stimulating factor and recombinant c-interferon: toxicity, monocytosis, and clinical effects. Cancer Res. 1994; 54:4084–90.

[47] Ulich T, del Castillo J, Watson L, Yin S and Garnick M. In vivo hematologic effects of recombinant human macrophage colony-stimulating factor. Blood. 1990; 75:846–50.

[48] Ryan GR, Dai XM, Dominguez MG, Tong W, Chuan F, Chisholm O, Russell RG, Pollard JW and Stanley ER. Rescue of the colony-stimulating factor 1 (CSF-1)-nullizygous mouse (Csf1(op)/Csf1(op)) phenotype with a CSF-1 transgene and identification of sites of local CSF-1 synthesis. Blood. 2001; 98:74–84.

[49] Lagasse E and Weissman IL. Enforced expression of Bcl-2 in monocytes rescues macrophages and partially reverses osteopetrosis in op/op mice. Cell. 1997; 89:1021–31.

[50] Burgess AW and Metcalf D. The nature and action of granulocyte–macrophage colony stimulating factors. Blood. 1980; 56:947–58.

[51] Gasson J. Molecular physiology of granulocyte–macrophage colony stimulating factor. Blood. 1991; 77:1131–45.

[52] Stanley E, Lieschke GJ, Grail D, Metcalf D, Hodgson G, Gall JA, Maher DW, Cebon J, Sinickas V and Dunn AR. Granulocyte/macrophage colony-stimulating factor-deficient mice show no major perturbation of hematopoiesis but develop a characteristic pulmonary pathology. Proc Natl Acad Sci. 1994; 91:5592–6.

[53] Sallusto F and Lanzavecchia A. Efficient presentation of soluble antigen by cultured human dendritic cells is maintained by granulocyte/macrophage colony-stimulating factor plus interleukin 4 and down-regulated by tumor necrosis factor alpha. J Exp Med. 1994; 179(4):1109–18.

[54] Caux C, Dezutter-Dambuyant C, Schmitt D and Banchereau J. GM-CSF and TNF-alpha cooperate in the generation of dendritic Langerhans cells. Nature. 1992; 360(6401):258–61.

[55] Jenkins SJ, Ruckerl D, Thomas GD, Hewitson JP, Duncan S, Brombacher F, Maizels RM, Hume DA and Allen JE. IL-4 directly signals tissue-resident macrophages to proliferate beyond homeostatic levels controlled by CSF-1. J Exp Med. 2013; 210:2477–91.

[56] Jenkins SJ, Ruckerl D, Cook PC, Jones LH, Finkelman FD, van Rooijen N, MacDonald AS and Allen JE. Local macrophage proliferation, rather than recruitment from the blood, is a signature of TH2 inflammation. Science. 2011; 332:1284–8.

[57] Bunting KD, Yu WM, Bradley HL, Haviernikova E, Kelly-Welch AE, Keegan AD and Qu CK. Increased numbers of committed myeloid progenitors but not primitive hematopoietic stem/progenitors in mice lacking STAT6 expression. J Leukoc Biol. 2004; 76:484–90.

[58] Verreck FAW, de Boer T, Langenberg DML, Hoeve MA, Kramer M, Vaisberg E, Kastelein R, Kolk A, de Waal-Malefyt R and Ottenhoff THM. Human IL-23-producing type 1 macrophages promote but IL-10-producing type 2 macrophages subvert immunity to (myco)bacteria. Proc Natl Acad Sci USA. 2004; 101:4560–5.

[59] Fischer HG, Frosch S, Reske K and Reske-Kunz AB. Granulocyte–macrophage colony-stimulating factor activates macrophages derived from bone marrow cultures to synthesis of MHC class II molecules and to augmented antigen presentation function. J Immunol. 1988; 141:3882–8.

[60] Martinez FO, Gordon S, Locati M and Mantovani A. Transcriptional profiling of the human monocyte-to-macrophage differentiation and polarization: new molecules and patterns of gene expression. J Immunol. 2006; 177:7303–11.

[61] Krausgruber T, Blazek K, Smallie T, Alzabin S, Lockstone H, Sahgal N, Hussell T, Feldmann M and Udalova IA. IRF5 promotes inflammatory macrophage polarization and TH1–TH17 responses. Nat Immunol. 2011; 12:231–8.

Chapter 2

Dendritic Cells: Location, Function, and Clinical Implications

Andrés Castell-Rodríguez, Gabriela Piñón-Zárate, Miguel Herrera-Enríquez, Katia Jarquín-Yáñez and Iliana Medina-Solares

Additional information is available at the end of the chapter

http://dx.doi.org/10.5772/intechopen.68352

Abstract

Dendritic cells (DCs) are antigen-presenting cells derived from bone marrow precursors and form a widely distributed cellular system throughout the body. DCs exert immune-surveillance for exogenous and endogenous antigens and the later activation of naive T lymphocytes giving rise to various immunological responses. Different growth factors and cytokines can modulate the differentiation and function of DCs, GM-CSF, M-CSF, Flt3, and TGF-β, resulting in a large variety of DCs with different functional abilities. Thus, DCs are classified as plasmacytoid DCs (pDCs), conventional DCs (cDCs), and DCs derived from monocytes (mDCs). Functionally, the cDCs may be divided into two states: immature and mature. Immature DCs are specialist in uptaking and processing antigens; in contrast, mature DCs are professional in antigen presentation. It has been observed that immature cDCs can induce immune tolerance while mature cDCs may induce Th2 or Th1 immune responses. It is worth noting that different subpopulations of DCs have the ability to secrete different cytokine patterns, resulting in the induction of different immunological responses. Furthermore DCs are involved in the pathophysiology of several diseases such as contact hypersensitivity, autoimmune diseases, or cancer, but they can also be used as therapeutic tools in these conditions.

Keywords: dendritic cells, immunotherapy, cancer, autoimmune diseases

1. Introduction

Dendritic cells (DCs) are antigen-presenting cells, characterized by a distinctive morphology and expression of markers such as CD11c and major histocompatibility complex class II molecules (MHCII). In addition, DCs can recognize pathogens, tissue damage signals, and tumor antigens and then migrate to the secondary lymphoid organs where they present antigens and activate T lymphocytes. DCs may induce the development of diverse immunological responses, either Th1, Th2, Treg, or Th17. There is a great variety of DCs with different phenotypes and localizations that form a cellular system distributed throughout the body and that is responsible for immune-surveillance. DCs are classified into conventional DCs (cDCs), plasmacytoids (pDCs), and DCs derived from monocytes (mDCs) [1, 2].

DCs are involved in many diseases, for example, contact hypersensitivity and autoimmune diseases, so intensive research is underway with the purpose of finding alternatives to induce the secretion of tolerogenic cytokines to decrease the activity of DCs in this type of pathologies [3, 4]. On the other hand, DCs have an important role in cancer. It has been observed that tumor cells may inhibit the maturation of DCs and induce the modification of their phenotype to provoke a Th17 or Treg response, which favors the proliferation of tumor cells. In addition, DCs are used as a promising alternative in cancer immunotherapy. To date, only one DC-based vaccine is available clinically; therefore, the study of immunomodulatory molecules that increase the maturation of DCs for their subsequent use in antitumor immunotherapy is underway [4, 5].

In the present chapter, the origin, phenotype of DCs precursors, and the description of the subpopulations located in the organism will be reviewed. Also, we analyze the different functional states of DCs and their relationship to the secreted cytokine pattern. Finally, we consider the role of DCs in some pathologies.

2. Dendritic cells biology

2.1. Origin and differentiation

2.1.1. Cytokines in DCs differentiation

DCs originate from hematopoietic precursor cells located in the bone marrow. Years ago, it was thought that DCs could have a lymphoid or a myeloid origin; then, after some experiments realized in 2007, it was found that DCs may originate from the common myeloid progenitor (CMP) and from the common lymphoid progenitor (CLP), giving rise to classical or conventional CDs, as well as plasmacytoid CDs [6]. It is important to note that key growth factors are needed for DC differentiations, such as Flt3L, granulocyte macrophage colony-stimulating factor (GM-CSF), and M-CSF [7] (**Figure 1**).

Among the different growth factors involved in DCs differentiation, the most important is Flt3-L, where the receptor is Flt3 (Fms-like tyrosine kinase 3), a receptor of a protein tyrosine kinase located especially in DCs precursor in bone marrow, so it has been proposed that Flt3-L is involved in the differentiation of cDCs and pDCs (**Figure 1**). It has also been suggested that Flt3-L/Flt3 regulates the maintenance and development of DCs in lymphoid and mucosal organs [8], as Flt3-L is sufficient for the differentiation of pDCs and cDCs from precursor

http://dx.doi.org/10.5772/intechopen.68352

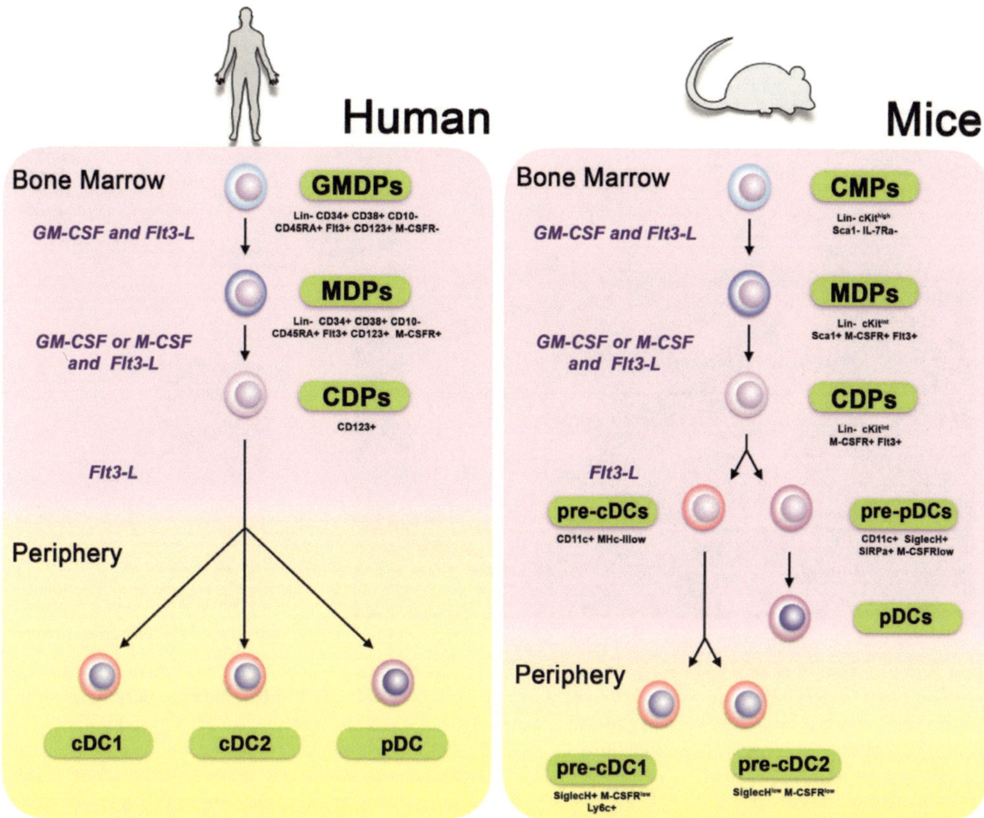

Figure 1. Differentiation of DCs in human and mouse. In human, three DCs precursors are recognized: GMDPs, MDPs, and CDPs. As the cells differentiate, they acquire different phenotype. It is accepted that under the influence of Flt3-L, cDC1, cDC2, and pDCs originate from CDPs. In mouse, it has been shown that there are several precursors: CMPs, MDPs, and CDPs. The latter differentiate into pre-cDCs and pre-pDCs. The pre-cDCs differentiate toward pre-cDC1 and pre-cDC2 giving rise to the cDC1 and cDC2, respectively. The pre-pDCs differentiate into pDCs. In the figure the phenotype of each cell and the cytokines involved in the differentiation process such as cell myeloid progenitors (CMPs), macrophages and dendritic cells progenitors (MDPs), common myeloid progenitors (CDPs), granulocytes, macrophages and DCs progenitors (GMDPs), pre-conventional dendritic cells (pre-cDCs), pre-plasmacytoid dendritic cells (pre-pDCs), pre-conventional dendritic cells 1 (pre-cDC1), pre-conventional dendritic cells 2 (pre-cDC2), conventional dendritic cells 1 (cDC1), conventional dendritic cells 2 (cDC2), plasmacytoid dendritic cells (pDCs) has been placed.

cells with various phenotypes *in vitro*, and when its expression is forced. In addition, Flt3-L deficient mice have shown only 10% of the pDCs and cDCs that are normally located in wild type, besides the administration of Flt3-L to those mice restored the levels of pDCs and cDCs, while the administration of Flt3-L to wild-type mice increased the levels of pDCs and cDCs in spleen [7, 9, 10].

Other important cytokine is granulocyte and macrophage colony-stimulating factor (**Figure 1**). It has been observed that it can induce the differentiation of DCs *in vitro* and *in vivo* (**Figure 2**); however, GM-CSF-deficient mice show normal levels of resident DCs of lymphoid organs, although there were some alterations in the levels of resident mucous or migratory DCs. So, it is believed that GM-CSF is not related to the differentiation of DCs in the steady state, but

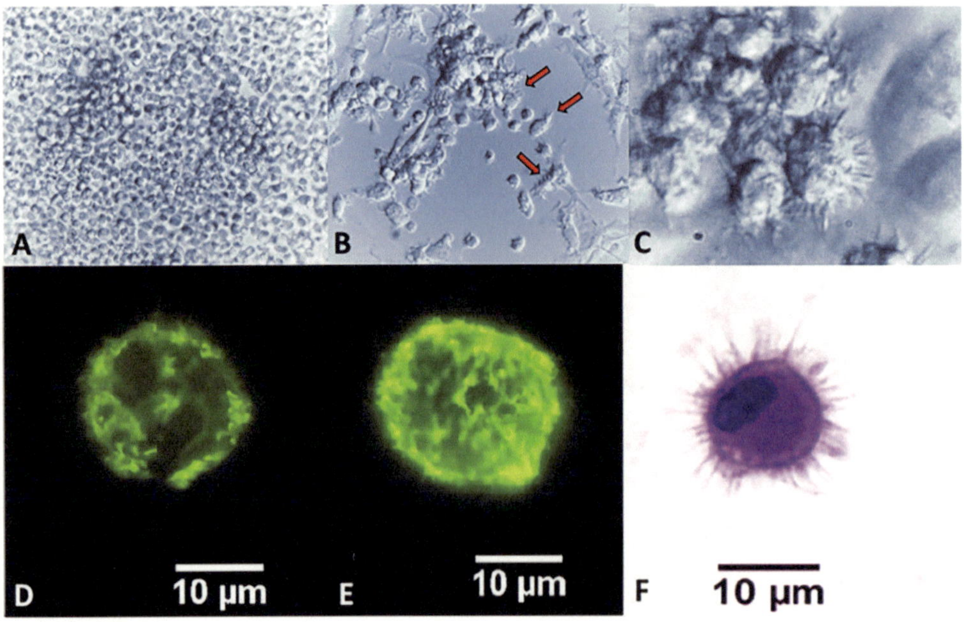

Figure 2. Differentiation of DCs from bone marrow precursors. The figure shows the differentiation of DCs from bone marrow precursor. (A) Culture of bone marrow cells at 24 h with GM-CSF. (B) and (C) The culture of bone marrow precursor cells after 6 days of culture with GM-CSF. The presence of poorly adherent cells with a great number of long and thin extensions is observed. (D) An immature DC MHCII positive is shown after 6 days of culture of bone marrow precursor cells with GM-CSF. (E) MHCII expression in DCs, after culturing for 2 h in the presence of LPS, a large increase in MHCII expression is observed. (F) A large number of extensions are observed in a DC stained with toluidine blue. The arrows point to DCs.

in the replenishment of DCs in non-lymphoid organs. In spite of the above, GM-CSF has been widely used in the differentiation of DCs *in vitro* that are subsequently used for therapeutic purposes [11, 12].

On the other hand, another cytokine involved in DCs differentiation is macrophage colony-stimulating factor (**Figure 1**). M-CSF is involved in DCs differentiation from monocytes and is very important for the differentiation of pDCs from certain MCSFR + cell populations in bone marrow. Nevertheless, knockout mice for M-CSF and its receptor did not show changes in DC levels in lymphoid organs, although there were decreased levels of monocytes and Langerhans cells (LCs) [13]. After all, now Flt3-L is considered as the most important cytokine in DCs development; nonetheless, M-CSF and GM-CSF are also relevant cytokines in DCs development and activation in non-lymphoid tissues [4, 13].

2.1.2. DCs precursors

The differentiation of DCs is carried out from various cell progenitor populations located in bone marrow (**Figure 1**). Multiple experiments have been conducted in order to characterize the different populations that can give rise to DCs, macrophages, or lymphocytes. These experiments include the isolation of cell populations by flow cytometry and the later treatment with Flt3-L, M-CSF, and GM-CSF or cultivated with stromal cells producing these cytokines

[8]. As a result, the first cell population with potential to differentiate into DCs, macrophages, monocytes, and polymorphonuclear cells was described and named cell myeloid progenitor (CMP), characterized by localizing in bone marrow and showing a Lin− c-Kit-high Sca1− IL-7Ralpha− phenotype. The CMP differentiation potential was evidenced when polymorphonuclear cells, macrophages, and DCs were obtained after CMPs were cultured with GM-CSF and Flt-3L-producing stromal cells [14]. Later, CMPs lose their potential to differentiate into granulocytes when initiated with the expression of M-CSFR. These progenitor cells are called macrophages and dendritic cell progenitors (MDPs), characterized by the phenotype Lin− Sca1− M-CSFR+ Flt3+ c Kit int CX3CR1+. The capacity of differentiation of the MDPs was evaluated by *in vitro* assays, where macrophages and DCs were obtained when MDPs were cultivated in the presence of M-CSF or GM-CSF. *In vivo* assays in irradiated mice showed that the inoculation of MDPs was directly involved in the differentiation of DCs and macrophages especially in lymphoid organs [13, 14].

Then, MDPs begin to decrease the c-Kit expression, which is indicative of differentiation into common dendritic cell progenitors (CDPs), characterized by the expression of the phenotype Lin− cKit^{int}, Flt3+ M-CSFR+. CDPs have the ability to differentiate into cDCs and pDCs with different phenotypes. So, when CDPs are cultivated in the presence of Flt3-L, a cell population CD11c+ MHCII+ is obtained; whereas, when CDPs are treated with GM-CSF a different cell population is obtained, since it shows the phenotype CD11c+ CD11b+ MHCII+. Also, when CDPs are treated with GM-CSF and Flt3-L cDCs and pDCs are acquired. *In vivo*, the potential of CDPs was evident when their inoculation in irradiated mice showed that CDPs were directly involved in the differentiation of CD11c+ CD8+ and CD11c+ CD8− cDCs and CD11c+B220+ pDCs. In conclusion, CDPs have the potential to differentiate just to pDCs and cDCs [13, 15].

CDPs have the potential to differentiate to Pre-pDCs and Pre-cDCs (pre-cDCs1 and pre-cDCs2). Pre-pDCs are characterized by the low expression of M-CSFR low [1], while it has been reported that Pre-cDCs is characterized by the expression of CD11c, Siglec-H, SIRPa low, and MHCII int. Pre-cDCs can be differentiated into Pre-cDC1s and Pre-cDC2s cells. The Pre-DC1s cells are known by decreasing the expression of M-CSFR, Siglec-H, and Ly6c. Ly6c is a monocyte marker. In the case of Pre-cDC2s, they maintain the expression of M-CSFR and Ly6c, but decrease the expression of Kit and Siglec-H. It is important to mention that Pre-DC1s, Pre-DC2s, and pDCs are located in the periphery, such as blood or lymphoid organs, whereas Pre-cDCs, Pre-pDCs, DCP, MDP, and CMP cells are located in the bone marrow [10, 16].

On the other hand, the DCs differentiation in human is a little different from its counterpart in mice (**Figure 1**). The cell with potential to differentiate into granulocyte, macrophage, and DCs is named granulocytes, macrophages, and DCs progenitor (GMDPs). This population is located in the bone marrow and may have the following phenotype: Lin− CD34+ CD38+ CD10− CD45RA+ Flt3+ CD123+ M-CSFR-. When these cells initiate the expression of M-CSFR, the phenotype changes and they are called macrophages and DCs progenitor, population with the capacity of differentiation to macrophages and DCs. Consequently, MDPs increase the expression of CD123, so they acquire the ability to differentiate just to DCs (pDCs and cDCs), so this cell population is called common DC progenitors (CDPs) [10] (**Figure 1**).

2.2. Dendritic cells subsets

2.2.1. Location

There is a great variety of DCs with different phenotypes and location. In general, DCs have been divided into conventional, plasmacytoid, and monocyte-derived [1]. The cDCs can be divided into cDC1s and cDC2s. The cDC1s are characterized by being CD8+ CD103+ in mouse and BDCA3+ (CD141+) in human. CDC2s phenotype is CD11b+ CD4+ CD8− in mouse and are BDCA1+ (CD1c+) in human. The plasmacytoid pDCs are positive for B220, mPDCA1 and Siglec-h in mice, while in humans they are BDCA4+ and BDCA2+ [17]. Another group of DCs derived from monocytes (mDCs) appears only when there is an inflammation. Langerhans cells, normal residents of the epidermis and epithelia, are not considered on the same lineage of the DCs mentioned above, since they originate from precursor cells that migrated to the skin before birth and differentiated into LCs during the first week of life [18].

In relation to the origin of the DCs, they all differ from bone marrow progenitor cells that have, as their common denominator, the expression of Flt3 and sometimes M-CSFR [19]. DCs are more numerous in lymphoid organs and epithelia. In addition, DCs can express various molecular markers depending on their location. Thus, pDCs, CD1s, and CD2s can be observed in different tissues of the organism [20]. **Figure 3** shows to which cluster of cDCs each cell belongs. It is necessary to consider the phenotype and particular location of DCs in relation to their function on that tissue. For example, the degree of maturation of DCs in lymphoid organs is different from that of DCs in other tissues, since DCs are sentinel cells responsible for the recognition of pathogens and signals of tissue damage, which induces their migration to lymphoid organs to carry out the activation of different subsets of T, natural killer (NK), NKT, and B lymphocytes. It has also been studied and analyzed for a long time that the inflammatory or tolerogenic microenvironment induced by the cytokines present in tissues is essential in the determination of the functions that DCs can have [17].

It is important to know the types of DCs located in the organism, as well as the cytokines involved in its activation, so the following explains the different types of DCs located in lymphoid organs, skin, gut, and blood (**Figure 4**).

2.2.1.1. DCs in lymphoid organs

2.2.1.1.1. Lymph nodes

In the lymph nodes, there are several subsets of DCs, one of them are the CD103+ migratory cDCs from peripheral tissues and generally exhibit a mature phenotype characterized by an increase in MHCII, CD80, CD86, and CD40. There are also two classes of resident DCs: CD8+, CD4+, or CD11b+, which possess an immature phenotype, unless there is an inflammatory environment in the lymph node. Also, the presence of CD141+ and CD1a+ DCs, reminiscent of the population of cells with the same marker in dermis, has been observed; therefore, these cells are considered as migratory [1, 20].

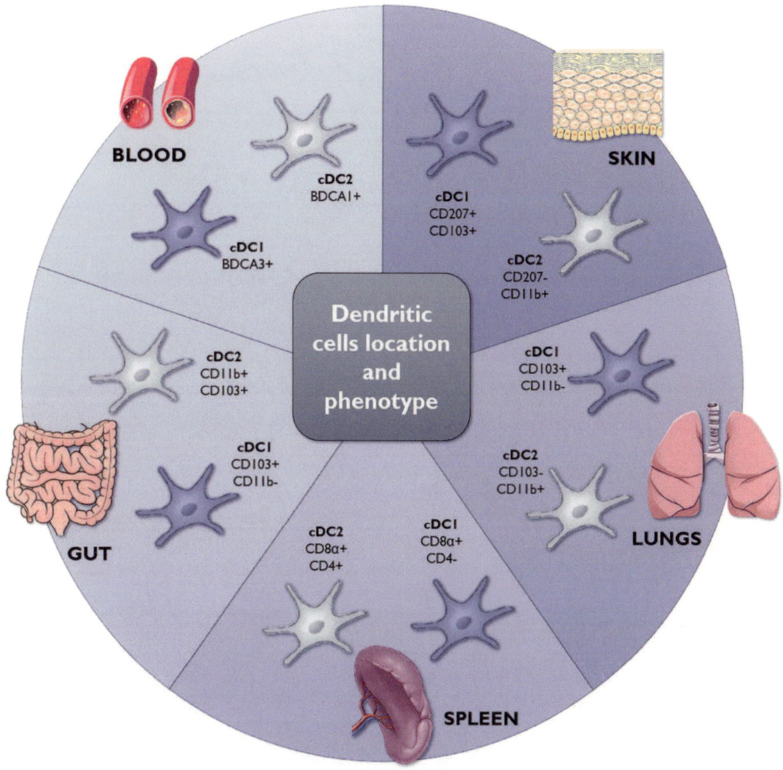

Figure 3. Dendritic cells location and phenotype. The cDCs (cDC1 and cDC2) may be located in lymphoid organs, blood, and mucous membranes. In lymphoid organs, the cDC1 (CD8+ CD4−) and cDC2 (CD8+ CD4+) are located. In mucoses such as respiratory tract and digestive tract, cDC1 (CD103+ CD11b−) and cDC2 (CD103+ CD11b+ or CD103− CD11b+) are also found. In blood, the cDC1 are BDCA3+ and the cDC2 express BDCA1+. In skin, the cDC1s are characterized by the expression of CD207+ CD103+, and the cDC2 for the expression of CD207− CD11b+.

2.2.1.1.2. Spleen

In the spleen, all DCs are CD8+ and are approximately 20% of the total spleen cells. DCs are classified into subsets according to CD11b marker expression. A subset is CD11b$^{low/-}$ DCs and shows an immature phenotype (MHCII^{low} CD80$^{low/-}$ CD86$^{low/-}$ CD40$^{low/-}$), proliferates in the presence of Flt3L, and expresses molecules such as CD205, CD207, and Clec9a. CD11+ DCs subsets are divided into DCs expressing high or low levels of the endothelial cell-specific adhesion molecule (ESAM). These two classes of DCs also proliferate in the presence of Flt3L and are CD4+ (ESAM) [21].

2.2.1.1.3. Thymus

In the thymus, there are at least three subsets of DCs: CD8+ cDCs (50%), Sirpα+ cDCs (20%), and pDCs (30%) [20]. CD8+ cDcS is likely to be derived from specific precursor cells. In this regard, studies have been investigated using the reporter of IL-7 receptor,

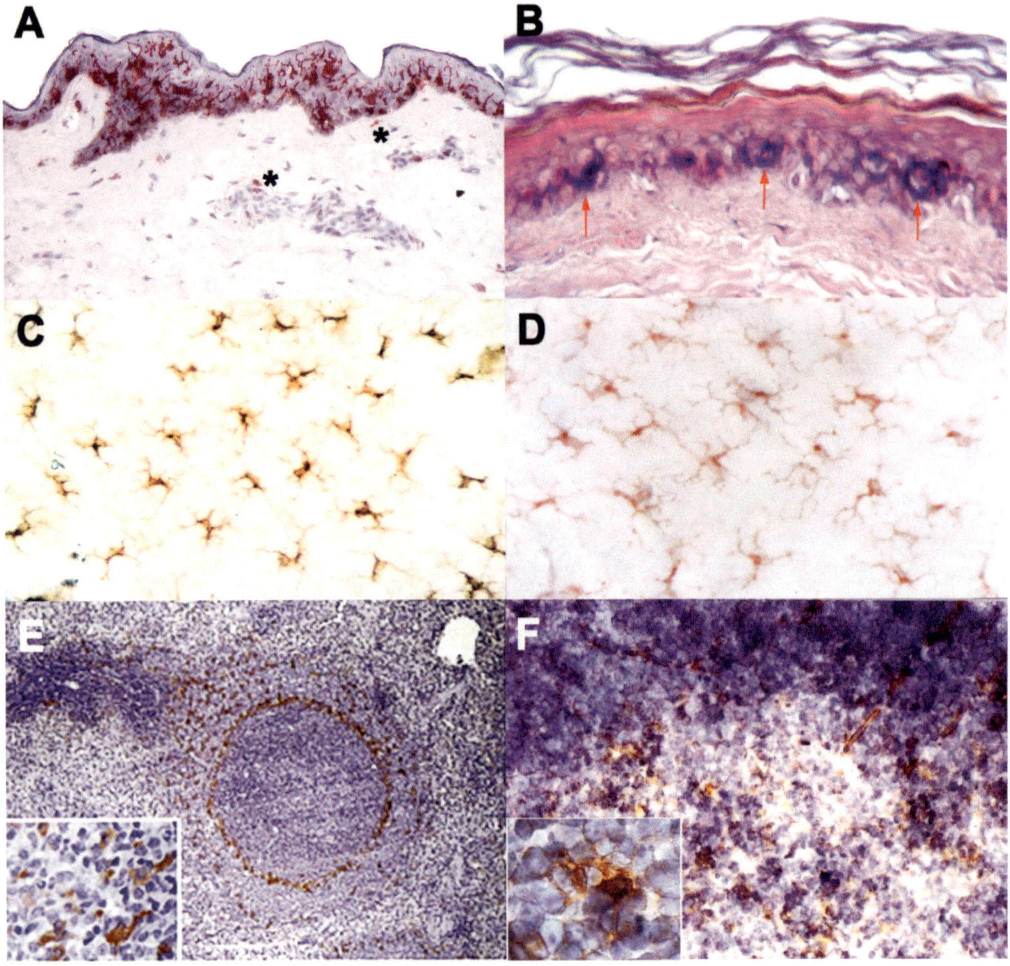

Figure 4. DCs at different locations. (A) and (B) human skin sections showing epidermal LCs positive for Langerin and CD1a, respectively. Arrows in (B) point to basal DCs. In (A), a few Langerin-positive cells (asterisks) are observed in the dermis. (C) and (D) Epidermal sheets of mouse skin with LCs positive for MHCII and CD205, respectively. In (E), a histological section of spleen showing Fascin-positive DCs is depicted. DCs are located in the T-dependent zone of the white pulp. In the thymus (F), a large amount of CD205-positive DCs is observed at the corticomedullary border.

which is a characteristic marker of lymphoid lineage, and of CD207, which is characteristic of CD8+ cDCs, and it has been found that only CD207 was expressed in thymic cDCs [22]. Using a new strategy named retroviral barcoding, it was determined that cDCs have a great similarity to spleen DCs and progenitors of bone marrow DCs [1]. Unlike CD8+ DCs, Sirpα+ DCs and pDCs develop extrathymically and are home to the thymus at steady state. Thymic homing of Sirpα+ DCs is dependent on a CCR2-mediated chemotaxis while pDC homing is dependent on CCR9 [23]. Both DC subsets are home to the thymus through blood vessels, but the specific tissues that originated from have not been comprehensively determined.

2.2.1.2. Blood

Multiple cell lines can be localized in the blood, such as granulocytes, monocytes, and lymphocytes, and to study blood DCs, several lineage markers (Lin), such as CD3, CD19, CD14, CD20, and CD56, are used to separate populations of DCs by means of flow cytometry assays [24]. Thus, populations of cDCs and pDCs can be identified in blood as they are Lin−. pDCs are characterized by expressing MHCII, BDCA2, and BDCA4, while the cDCs express MHCII and CD11c. Both types of DCs are negative for Lin markers. The cDCs divide into two subtypes, BDCA1 (CD1c) or CD141 (BDCA3) cells [25, 26].

2.2.1.3. Skin

In epidermis and dermis, different types of DCs can be found. In the epidermis, LCs constitute 2–4% and are characterized by expressing high concentrations of Langerin (CD207), CD45, and low concentrations of CD11c and MHCII. In humans, the expression of CD1a has also been observed, but not in mice. Unlike the other DCs, the differentiation of LCs is independent of Flt3; however, they are dependent for their development of Csf-1R, which also induces macrophage differentiation, M-CSF, in addition to chemokines CCL2 and CCL20 [18]. Langerhans cells were considered to be bone marrow dependent; however, it has been observed that LCs may have two distinct embryonic origins: the fetal liver and the yolk sac. In the mouse dermis, two populations of DCs, the CD103+ and CD8α+, have been observed, whose origin is based on the precursor of DCs positive for CLEC9A. It has been observed that when these cells are CD24^{low}, CD11b^{low}, and Sirpα+, they are involved in the development of Th2 and Th17 responses [27]. In humans, LCs have a phenotype very similar to that of mice, and they may respond to IL-15. On the other hand, in the dermis are several subsets of DCs: CD14+ CD1a− DCs, CD14− CD1a+ DCs, and 6-sulpho LacNAc+ DCs [28]. The CD14+ DCs are poor activators of CD8+ T cells in contrast to CD14− DCs. The subset CD141+ DCs is extremely successful in the activation of CD4+ T lymphocytes. The population of pDCs located in the dermis is very low; however, in inflammatory skin diseases such as psoriasis or lupus erythematosus, an increase of this type of skin cells has been observed [29].

2.2.1.4. Gut

DCs in the intestine are located in the lamina propria of the intestinal mucosa, especially in the Peyer's patches of the small intestine. These cells are usually CD103+, CD8+, and CD207+, express low concentrations of MHCII, and have been observed to proliferate when there are high concentrations of Flt3. There is a second type of DCs that are also located in the lamina propria, but which express the markers CD103 and CD11b, although CD103 is expressed in low levels. These types of DCs can also be localized in the muscular layer of the digestive tract, so they may be confused with CD11b+ macrophages [30].

2.2.2. Cytokine production

As previously mentioned, the DC differentiation is a process occurring in bone marrow. It depends on key cytokines (Flt3-L, GM-CSF, and M-CSF) and different cell precursors such as the common myeloid progenitor and the common lymphoid progenitor resulting in the obtaining of classical (cDCs) and plasmacytoid DCs (pDCs [17, 18, 31, 32]. As a result of this process, different DC populations not only acquire different phenotypes but also colonize different tissues and perform different functions [31]. However, when precursors of dendritic cells are differentiated in the presence of different factors such as GM-CSF and tumor necrosis factor-α (TNF-α), at least two CDs populations give rise, one characterized by the expression of CD1a+/E-cadherin+ and another characterized by the expression of CD14+/CD68+. Both populations shared some characteristics, such as the secretion of some cytokines (IL-1, IL-1, IL-6, IL-7, IL-12, IL-15, IL-18, TNF-, TGF-, M-CSF, and GM-CSF). However, when these cells are treated with CD40 ligands, DCs acquire the ability to produce IL-10 and IL-13 [31].

The progression in the maturation/activation state of the different CDs populations involves not only changes in the expression of the receptors present in the cell membrane but also their ability to interact with the extra cellular environment and with other cells. In this sense, both immature CDs in lymphoid and mucosal tissue and differentiated CDs *in vitro* are characterized by (1) having a weak antigenic presentation capacity, since DCs express low levels of MHC-II molecules, and co-stimulatory molecules (CD40, CD80, and CD86), where expression increases when DCs are exposed to maturation stimulus such as CD40L or IFN-γ; (2) having a high expression of tissue damage receptors such as CD36 and Toll-like receptors [26]; (3) having a high expression of molecules involved in the capture of antigens of different chemical origin, such as FcγRI, CD1, CD205, CD207, CD209, and CLEC-9 [33–37], receptors involved in antigenic internalization and in the release of intracellular signals, promoting greater expression of adhesion molecules [38, 39]; (4) changes in the production of cytokines after undergoing the maturation/activation process. Mature CDs produce differentially cytokines related to promote the different immune responses (Th1, Th2, Th17, and Treg).

In this section, we describe the patterns of cytokine production, produced by the different subsets of DCs.

2.2.2.1. Conventional DCs

Human cDCs differentiated from bone marrow precursors in the presence of GM-CSF and IL-4 differentially show not only the expression of mRNA but also the production and release of different cytokines depending on their maturation stage.

Immature DCs are characterized by having a phenotype CD11c+, CD86–, $MHCI^{low}$, $MHCII^{low}$, CD40–, $CD80^{low}$, $CD54^{low}$, OX40–, and CD8a–, whereas mature DCs are characterized by a phenotype CD11c+, CD83+, CD86+, $MHCI^{low}$, $MHCII^{high}$, CD40+, CD80+, CD54+, OX40+, and CD8a–. Both immature and mature DCs have different cytokine pattern secretion (**Table 1**) [17, 32].

It has been observed that the differential expression of cytokines is regulated not only according to the type of DCs but also by the activation pathway. lipopolysaccharide (LPS)-stimulated DCs have been shown to exhibit a positive regulation of IL-1α, IL-1β, and IL-6 and to a lesser degree of IL-15, TNF-α, and MIF. On the other hand, when DCs are stimulated with

Cytokines profile produced by cDCs					
Cytokine	**Immature DCS**	**Mature DCs**	**Activation path of mature DCs**		
			LPS	**Anti CD40**	**TNFα**
IL1a	High	Low	High	Low	Low
IL-1β	High	Low	High	Low	Low
IL-2	Negative	Negative	Negative	–	Médium
IL-4	Low	Medium	Medium	–	High
IL-6	Low	Medium	Low	Medium	Low
IL_d10	Low	Medium	Medium	Medium	Medium
IL-12	Low	High	High	High	High
IL-12 p35	Negative	High	High	Medium	Medium
IL-12 p40	Low	High	Medium	High	–
IL-12p70	Low	High	High	High	High
IL-13	Low	High	Low	Low	High
IL-15	Low	High	Medium	High	–
IL-18	Low	Medium	Low	Medium	–
IL-23	Low	High	High	Negative	–
MIF	High	High	High	High	–
IFN-γ	Low	Medium	Low	–	High
TGF-β whole	Low	Low	Negative	–	Low
TGF-β1	Low	Low	–	–	Medium
TGF-β2	Low	Low	–	–	–
TGF-β3	Low	Low	–	–	–
TNF-α	Low	High	High	Medium	Medium

Table 1. Cytokines secreted by immature DCs, mature and matured by different pathways.

anti-CD40 antibodies only discrete changes are observed in the levels of some cytokines, such as IL-6, IL-12p40, IL-15, and TNF-α, whereas IL-1α, IL-1β, IL-18, IFN-γ, TGFβ1-3, and MIF are not altered. This fact acquires relevance since those DCs that are stimulated via anti-CD40 may exhibit a phenotype of cDC1s or cDC2s being able to guide the immunological response to both TH1 and Th2. By contrast, DCs that are stimulated with LPS show a phenotype of cDC1s. This fact is due to a differential signal on the production of IL-23 which strongly interacts with IL-12 [24, 40].

This same pattern of differential activation has been observed in mature murine and canine DCs, stimulated with different types of signals, either with endogenous or with exogenous stimuli, where regardless of the type of stimulus, mature DCs show a phenotype with an increased expression of CD11c, IL-10β, IL-12p40, IL-12β, IL-12β, IL-12β, IL-12β, IL-12β, IL-13, and TNF-α, thus contributing to awakening a Th1-type response. In contrast, TNF-α-stimulated DCs show increased expression of IL-2, IL-4, IL-12p40, IL-13, TNF-α, TGF-β, IFN-γ, and MCP-2 promoting a Th2 response. This differential production of cytokines appears to be due to the involvement of IL-13 that acts similarly to IL-4, thus promoting this response Th2 [41, 42] (**Table 1**).

2.2.2.2. Tolerogenic DCs

Characteristically, some subsets of DCs of myeloid origin that modulate the antigen-specific adaptive immune response by presenting auto-peptides to CD4+ T cells in the presence of inhibitory signals, anti-inflammatory cytokines, or other molecules that promote regulatory T cell populations are also capable of inducing the deletion or clonal anergy of autoreactive T cells.

Some mechanisms of the generation of tolerogenic DCs involve stimulation with IL-10, TGF-β, IL-6, TNF-α or its combination [43–46], as well as weak stimulation with bacterial products like LPS [47], pharmaceutical drugs like dexamethasone [48], and inhibitors of cell signaling such as PKCi or CTLA4 [49, 50]. These cells acquire a tolerogenic activity characterized by an immature phenotype with weak expression of co-stimulatory molecules, but with a differential production of anti- and proinflammatory cytokines.

This production of cytokines by tolerogenic DCs is dependent on the microenvironment in which they are found. Thus, the presence of IL-10 promotes a decrease in IL-6, IL-12, and IL-23, as well as an increase in the release of TGF-β, PGE_2, and IL-10, leading to an increase in Treg cell populations. In contrast, in the presence of high concentrations of TGF-β, tolerogenic DCs show a high expression of the co-inhibitory molecules ILT4, PDL-1, and PDL-2 [51, 52]. The synergism of IL-10 and TGF-β promotes similar cytokine production in DCs, but DCs also show a high CCR7-dependent migratory capacity with low antigenic activity.

When there is an early exposure to IFN-γ, DCs are guided to a tolerogenic phenotype with a reduced endocytic capacity as well as weak expression of IL-12, IL-23, and TNF-α, an effect that is maintained even after receiving a second proinflammatory stimulation [53] (**Table 2**).

2.2.2.3. Plasmacytoid cells

Since their description, pDCs have produced a great controversy about their origin and function. Unlike other DCs, pDCs generation is controlled by the expression of the transcription factor E2-2 [54]. pDCs express CCR9, CD9, CD19, CD123, CD303, and CD304 molecules. They also express the BDCA2 receptor, and the histidine transporter Slc15a4, which facilitate the signaling of TLRs and the production of IFN and other cytokines [55]. In mice, the pDCs express PDCA1 and Siglec-H [56]. In their immature or inactive state, they have a similar appearance to plasmatic cells, lacking dendritic cytoplasmic projections, do not show an ability for uptake and present antigens and produce large amounts of IFN types I and III. However, when these cells are activated, they rapidly undergo a morphological and functional conversion similar to that of cDCs with a capacity to stimulate T cells [2].

Phenotype and cytokine production by tolerogenic DCs			
Mechanism	**Phenotype**	**Cytokine**	**Tolerance mechanism**
IL-10	Low expression of costimulatory molecules CD11c+, MHCII^{low}, CD80^{low}, and CD86^{low} Weak migratory capacity CCR7^{low}	Low secretion of IL-6, IL-12, and IL-23 High secretion of IL-10, PGE2, and TGF-β	Anergy of CD4+ T cells Induction of Treg cells
TGF-β	Low expression of costimulatory molecules CD11c+ MHCII^{low}, CD80^{low}, and CD86^{low} High expression of inhibitory molecules ILT4^{high} and PD-LI/2^{high}	Low secretion of Il-β, IL-6, and IL-12 e IL-23 High secretion of IL-10	Anergy of CD4+ T cells Induction of Treg cells Inhibition of the secretion of INFγ by CD4+ T cells
IL10 + TGF-β	Low expression of costimulatory molecules CD11c+ MHCHII^{low}, CD80^{low}, and CD86^{low} High migratory capacity CCR7^{high} Weak antigenic presentation activity	Low secretion of IL-6, IL-12, IL-18, and IL-23 High expression of IL-4, IL-5, PGE2, and TGF-β	Anergy of CD4+ T cells Promotion of stimulated T-cells-producing IL2^{low}, IFN-γ^{low} IL-10^{high}
Dex	Low expression of costimulatory molecules CD11c+, MHCII^{low}, CD80^{low}, and CD86^{low} High migratory capacity CCR7^{high} and CXCR4^{high}	Low secretion of IL-12, IL-23, and TNF-α High secretion of IL-10	Anergy of CD4+T cells Induction of Tr1 cells-producing IL-10
IFN-γ early exposition	Low expression of costimulatory molecules CDIIc+ MHCII^{low}, CD80^{low}, and CD86^{low} Weak endocitic capacity	Low secretion of IL-12	Induction of Treg cells CD127$^{-/low}$, CD25^{high}, and FoxP3+ Induction of Treg cells IL10+, TGF-β+, and FoxP3+

Table 2. Tolerogenic DCs activation pathways with their cytokine secretion profile and phenotype.

They are known to share with cDCs not only the same progenitor but also the dependence of some factors for their differentiation as the cytokine FMS-related tyrosine kinase 3 ligand (Flt3L) and interferon-regulating factor 8 (IRF8) [56]. Like other DCs, pDCs are deficient of lymphocytic lineage markers. When pDCs are activated by ligands of TLR7 and TLR9, they produce high amounts of IFNs types I and III, other cytokines such as IL-6 and IL-12 as well as chemokine ligands CCL3, CCL4, CCL5, CXCL9, CXCL10, and CXCL11 [57, 58]. The regulatory capacity of pDCs involves the expression of the indoleamine 2,3-dioxygenase (IDO) enzyme [52], a suboptimal presentation of antigens, and the induction of Treg cells [57, 58].

2.3. Processing and antigen presentation

DCs are capable of capturing and processing antigens very efficiently and for this they possess several molecules that have been identified and are discussed below. In general, two antigen-processing pathways have been defined, the endocytic pathway and the cytosolic pathway, through which exogenous and endogenous antigens are presented, respectively [59].

2.3.1. Exogenous antigens: endocytic way

Exogenous antigens, such as those derived from bacteria, are captured by immature DCs by means of endocytosis, phagocytosis, or both, through different molecules such as Fc receptors of IgG or lectins such as CD205, which guides their internalization into endocytic compartments with increasing acidity: slightly acidic early endosomes, moderately acidic endolysosomes, and very acidic late endolysosomes [60]. The late endolysosomes are very rich in MHCII and it is in these compartments where the antigens are degraded in polypeptides of 13–18 residues by some acidic proteases such as thiol and aspartyl cathepsins specific for the substrate [61, 62]. In these compartments, cathepsin degrades the invariant chain (li) bound to MHCII to a 24 amino acid peptide called the class II invariant chain peptide (CLIP), which occupies the cleavage of chains $\alpha 1$ and $\beta 1$ of MHCII. This degradation is regulated by the concentrations of cathepsin S and its inhibitor endogenous cystatin C. After the DCs have matured, cystatin C decreases and cathepsin S activity is increased, promoting the degradation of Ii toward CLIP [62, 63]. The cleavage of MHCII where CLIP is placed is the site that can occupy the processed antigens and accommodates peptides up to 30 amino acids in size. As the CLIP is occupying this cleft, it needs to be removed so that it can be occupied by degraded exogenous antigens [61]. This process is induced by human leukocyte antigen (HLA)-DM molecules, which structurally resemble MHCII and are not expressed on the cell surface of DCs, but act as a peptide exchanger, facilitating the capture of CLIP, leaving the cleft of MHC II free to be occupied by the degraded antigenic peptide, resulting in the stabilization of MHCII [64]. Finally, the MHCII/processed peptide complex is carried through transport vesicles to the plasma membrane where the peptide can be recognized by CD4+ T lymphocytes specific for the peptide antigen presented [65]. The overall process is shown in **Figure 5**.

2.3.2. Endogenous antigens: cytoplasmic way

Presentation of endogenous antigens by MHCI molecules is performed on all nucleated cells and involves the degradation of cytosolic proteins and the loading of the resulting peptides into newly synthesized MHCI within the rough endoplasmic reticulum [66]. It is worth noting that this antigen-processing route also processes viral proteins from infected cells and proteins from bacteria that were initially phagocytosed and processed into endosomes but escaped from them into the cytoplasm. All these proteins, located in the cytoplasm, are susceptible to be degraded by proteasomes [67]. The processing of cytoplasmic proteins begins when they are conjugated with several copies of ubiquitin which is recognized by proteasomes. The proteasomes are formed by four protein cylinders, two peripheral α rings, and two β central rings. The β rings have catalytic activity located in the $\beta 1$, $\beta 2$, and $\beta 3$ subunits. Proteasomes have a broad specificity of protein substrates and can generate a large variety of peptides capable of being presented by MHC class I molecules [66, 67]. DCs are highly efficient in the processing and presentation of cytosolic proteins because they possess constitutively di-ubiquitin, which has a tandem of key functional protein motifs, and proteasomes with a substrate specificity that allows peptides resulting from degradation of proteins have a large amount of hydrophobic

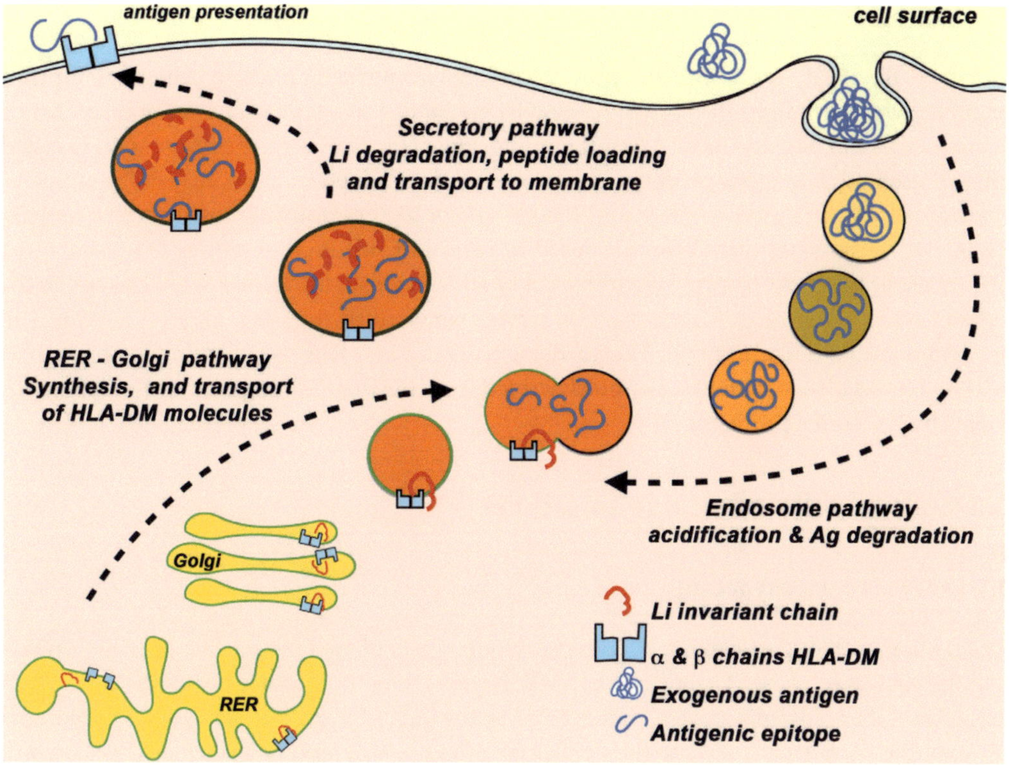

Figure 5. Exogenous antigens processing: endocytic way. Exogenous antigens are captured by immature DCs by endocytosis, phagocytosis, or both. Antigens are internalized into endocytic compartments where cathepsin degrades the invariant chain (li) bound to MHCII to a class II-invariant chain peptide (CLIP), which occupies the cleavage of MHCII. Then, CLIP is removed by HLA-DM molecules and the processed antigens occupy the space. Finally, the MHCII/processed peptide complex is carried through transport vesicles to the plasma membrane where the peptide can be recognized by CD4+ T lymphocytes.

or basic amino acids, which gives them a high affinity for MHC class I molecules [59, 68]. In particular, INF-γ and TNF-α, two proinflammatory cytokines, can induce a rapid increase of proteasomes in DCs, along with an increased expression of MHCI [69].

Peptides resulting from protein degradation are transported by an ATP-dependent process into the endoplasmic reticulum by a specific antigen-processing (TAP) transporter, which consists of two transmembrane proteins called TAP1 and TAP2 [67]. The transported peptides may have different lengths, but the transport is optimum for peptides of 8–16 amino acids [61]. Note that MHCIs are associated with TAP by means of a small protein called Tapasin, which retains MHCI in the endoplasmic reticulum until the peptide has conjugated to them. Inside the reticulum, the transported peptide is cut to a length of nine amino acids by a specific aminopeptidase in order to fit into the cleavage of MHCI [66]. When this happens, Tapasin releases the class I molecules coupled to the peptide antigen that can then be transported to the Golgi apparatus and from there to vesicles of transport to the plasma membrane of the cells where the antigenic peptides can be presented specifically to CD8+ T lymphocytes [59].

2.3.3. Cross-priming

DCs have the ability to capture and process proteins from virally infected cells or tumor cells and that, when processed through the endocytic pathway, can be presented not only to CD4+ T lymphocytes but also to CD8+ T virgin lymphocytes [60]. This type of presentation is called cross-presentation or cross-priming. This process is determined by the nature of the antigens, the way they have been captured, and the subsets of DCs performing the presentation [65]. Thus, two approaches have been proposed to carry out this type of antigenic presentation. The cytosolic pathway involves the transport of antigens from the lumen of endosomes to the cytosol where they can be processed by proteasomes until they are coupled to MHCI in the endoplasmic reticulum [69]. The vacuolar pathway involves the coupling in endosomes of class I molecules to antigenic peptides derived from the degradation of endocytic compartments by lysosomal proteases [70].

3. Dendritic cells: clinical implications

3.1. Delayed contact hypersensitivity

The pathophysiology of contact hypersensitivity consists of two phases: the induction phase and the challenge phase. The induction phase begins when the haptens penetrate the stratum corneum of the epidermis and are endocytosed by the LCs. LCs are then activated and migrated through the lymphatic vessels to the paracortex of regional lymph nodes, where they present the haptens in the context of MHCII to CD4+ T lymphocytes [71]. These activated T lymphocytes specific for these haptens are expanded clonally and finally reach the circulatory torrent. During this process, they express the cutaneous leukocyte antigen (CLA), with which they have the possibility to return preferentially to the skin through the high endothelium postcapillary veins [72]. The lymphocytes generated in this process are antigen-specific memory lymphocytes [73]. This phase lasts in the human between 10 and 15 days and has no clinical repercussions.

The challenge phase begins when haptens, which have already stimulated the induction phase, are brought into second contact with the skin. These haptens are endocytosed and presented by LCs, keratinocytes, or dermal DCs [74], which can present them to antigen-specific memory T lymphocytes located on the skin. Memory T lymphocytes activate CD8+ cytotoxic T lymphocytes which are the main effector cells in contact hypersensitivity. These lymphocytes secrete inflammatory cytokines and chemokines and induce apoptosis in keratinocytes [75]. Then, intense chemotaxis of different leukocytes is produced toward the skin resulting in a large inflammatory skin reaction [76]. Among the leukocytes that are also attracted are CD4+ Treg lymphocytes that modulate the inflammatory response. In humans, this phase occurs at 72 h and persists for a few days, after which it rapidly decreases by mechanisms mediated by CD4+Treg lymphocytes [72].

3.2. Autoimmune diseases

Throughout the development, the maturation of the adaptive immune system and during the induction of immune responses, B and T lymphocytes show a high rate of genetic recombination in the variable and hypervariable regions of the antigen receptors, so that the adaptive immune system has a wide variety of antigen receptors, being able to respond to virtually any type of molecule. Because of this phenomenon, there is a high probability that different self-antigens are recognized by the immune system, in addition to nonself antigens [1, 77]. To prevent the system from reacting against a self-antigen, autoreactive lymphocytes must be removed or trained as tolerant cells. Resident reticuloepithelial cells from cortex and marrow of the thymus perform a negative selection process to eliminate such autoreactive clones. In this sense, it has been demonstrated that thymic DCs are also actively involved in such negative selection processes, and more recently it has been shown that even peripheral DCs may migrate to the thymus and participate in this selection [1, 23]. This is highly significant as some populations of DCs are directly related to the development of autoimmune diseases, which has recently been shown in a study using transgenic mice transfected with diphtheria toxin A (DTA) coupled to a resistance cassette to neomycin which were crossed with CD11c-Cre mice.

In the progeny, the Cre complex removes the resistance cassette generating toxicity in CD11c+ cells, resulting in depletion of DCs including conventional, plasmacytoid, and LCs, which led to an increase in the frequency of CD4+ thymocytes and CD4+ lymphocytes in tissues together with the spontaneous development of multiorgan autoimmunity [78, 79]. On the other hand, the participation of immature DCs in the induction of Treg cells has been documented, where CD205 receptor stimulation led to a tolerant antigenic presentation, resulting in an increase of CD25+ CTLA-4 T cells, via ligands of co-stimulatory molecules such as CD28 and CD154, as well as a decrease in IL-2 production and CD4 [79, 80] T proliferation. Thus, immature DCs play a crucial role in the activation of Treg, not only to autoantigens but also against alloantigens, since it has been observed that the repeated stimulation of CD4+ T cells with immature allogeneic DCs in the absence of antigens leads to a differentiation toward Tregs cells [81].

On the other hand, it has been evidenced that in a state of non-inflammation (steady state), the tolerant response by the immature DCs depends strongly on the control of TGF-β1 [107]. LCs and bmDCs upregulate the expression of Axl, which belongs to the family of tyrosine kinase receptors, Tyro3, Axl Mer (TAM), which has the function of inhibiting the inflammatory response in DCs, in addition to participating in the elimination of apoptotic cells and the blockade of proinflammatory cytokine production, which together is essential for the maintenance of self-tolerance [27].

The participation of DCs in autoimmune processes has been controversial, since in different studies the ability of DCs to break tolerance and to induce autoimmune responses has been reported, and others have described the ability of DCs to preserve tolerance and avoid an autoimmune response. Thus, much of the controversy is due to the functional diversity of the different DCs populations, namely that while mature DCs can induce strong self-reactive responses, for example, in the central nervous system an amplification of experimental autoimmune encephalitis has been observed; it has also been observed that the use of immature DCs has the capacity to offer protection against the development of autoimmune reactions [81, 82].

Immature and tolerogenic DCs produce high levels of IL10, IL-2, and TGF-β, which effectively promotes the proliferation and activation of inducible regulatory T cells (iTreg), decreasing the autoimmune reaction; however, if the tolerance in different models cannot be restored, possibly it is due to the activity of CD220+ B cells that potently modulate Th17 responses, maintaining the proinflammatory state [79].

The use of DCs as a therapeutic tool in autoimmune reactions has to do not only with their ability to produce tolerance-inducing cytokines such as IL-10 and TGF but also with their biological capabilities such as the expression of molecules involved in the antigen presentation. For example, two populations of IL-10 modulated DCs (IL10DC) having a $CD83^{High}$, CCR7+, or $CD83^{low}$ CCR7-phenotype were recently compared. Assays suppression effector T cells showed that iTreg from the $CD83^{High}$ IL-10DCs induced greater suppression than the population of iTreg from the $CD83^{low}$ IL-10DCs, and had a higher migratory capacity to lymph nodes, suggesting that they are a good therapeutic candidate [52].

In addition to tolerogenic DCs, other DCs are involved in the modulation of autoimmune responses. Thus, other populations of DCs such as plasmacytoids have been evaluated. In a model of arthritis induced by methylated bovine serum albumin (mBSA), it is known that IFN-α prevents the inflammatory process, pDCs function was assessed in relation to TGF-β and IDO. IFN-α was found to increase the expression of IDO1 and the corresponding TGF-β signaling in the pDCs. Likewise, it was also observed that the depletion of the pDCs, either during the sensitization phase or already initiated the arthritic response, eliminates the protective effect of IFN-α. In addition, this same abrogating effect of IFN-α activity was observed when TGF-β signaling was blocked, but exclusively in the signaling phase, implying that this IDO1/TGF-β protection pathway is dependent on anti-inflammatory programs, while responses to restimulation are dependent on the participation of the pDCs [83].

As previously mentioned, TLR7 and TLR9 play an important role in the biology of pDCs, which also involves them in autoimmune responses. In a murine model deficient mice of the Gfi1-transcriptional repressor, which modulates myeloid and lymphoid differentiation, show spontaneous autoimmunity like lupus, including high levels of IgM and IgG2a, autoantibodies against RNA and DNA, as well as an increased frequency of plasmoblasts and germinal centers. In contrast, Gif1 mice do not show this phenotype, but interestingly they show an increase in TLR7-dependent DCs activation, where stimulated DCs produce increased amounts of TNF-α, IL-6, and IFN-β as well as an increase in phosphorylation of the transcription factors NF-κB and IRF7, suggesting the control of the IFN-I-signaling pathway, so that apparently the negative regulation of TLR7 in DCs prevents the spontaneous development of lupus [81].

3.3. Cancer

Tumor cells have mechanisms to evade the immune system such as the decreased expression of class I molecules, the release of tolerogenic cytokines such as TGF-β and IL-10, as well as the induction of lymphocyte death. Generally, in the tumor stroma Treg cells, macrophages type 2, mast cells, inhibitory myeloid cells, and neutrophils may secrete cytokines that help the growth of the tumor; also, the formation of free radicals may contribute to increase the mutation rate in tumor cells [84]. In the stroma, there are also immature DCs that can induce the activation of Tregs tumor antigen-specific antigen lymphocytes, which may be involved with increased tumor growth [85]. In addition, DCs have been isolated from patients with metastases or with advanced stages of the disease and it has been shown that DCs express co-inhibitory molecules such as PD-L1, arginase, and IDO, and produce TGF-β, IL-10, and prostaglandins E2, resulting in an inhibition of T lymphocytes. It is worth noting that the use of immunostimulators can inhibit this suppression effect induced by DCs [86, 87]. In some patients, small foci of extratumoral lymphoid tissue known as tertiary lymphoid tissue may be localized and in them it is common to find memory T lymphocytes and naive T lymphocytes, in addition to mature DCs. When DCs and T lymphocytes have been isolated from this tissue, the development of a Th1 response has been observed in addition to the increased survival of patients with cancer. It is important to emphasize that this lymphoid tissue is usually observed in the early stages of the disease.

3.3.1. *Antitumoral immunotherapy*

DCs can be used in antitumor immunotherapy to induce the development of effective immunological responses that decrease the size of the tumor mass and increase survival. CD8+ T lymphocytes and NK cells, through the release of perforins and granzymes or through the binding of FAS/FASL molecules, can induce the death of tumor cells. These lymphocytes may be activated by DCs that have presented antigens from a tumor in the lymph nodes closest to the tumor mass. Thus, DCs have been differentiated *in vitro* to be used as a type of adoptive immunotherapy in clinical protocols. There are multiple strategies that have been used with DCs as described below.

DCs derived from bone marrow precursor cells and DCs derived from monocytes have been used in clinical protocols, with the latter being the most used in immunotherapy against melanoma [4, 88]. Cytokines (IL-4, IL-15, and IFN-γ), TLR agonists such as nucleic acids (CpG), Imiquimod, LPS, monophosphoryl lipid A, BCG, as well as transfection of DCs with RNA, encoding cytokines, growth factors, and co-stimulatory molecules, have been used to mature DCs [89].

In relation to the antigens used, DCs treated with nucleic acids, whole tumor antigens, tumor lysates, and peptides have been used to carry out a specific antitumor response [8]. The clinical results have been variable, so DCs-based immunotherapy has been used in combination with the administration of antibodies, cytokines, and even radiotherapy and chemotherapy [90].

Regarding melanoma tumor antigens, several have been used to stimulate DCs to elicit a specific antitumor immunological response dependent on T CD8 lymphocytes, capable on inducing cell tumor death. In this sense, some of the antigens most used for antitumor immunotherapy against melanoma are MAGE proteins [91, 92], gp-100 [93], NY-ESO, and tyrosinase, among others. Also, in different clinical assays, DCs have been loaded with one or more tumor antigens, for example, DCs loaded with various melanoma-specific antigens (gp-100 and tyrosinase) were administered in patients with melanoma and had a regression success rate of 11% [94], whereas in another clinical study, in which the same antigens were used in conjunction with keyhole hemocyanin, 57% of those receiving the therapy showed no tumor growth and only 4% showed complete tumor regression [29].

The success of DCs loaded with proteins or with tumor peptides has been moderate and is generally because antigen-specific T lymphocyte proliferation is not high; however, DC-based immunotherapy has been more successful than other strategies (e.g., the use of peptide-based vaccines) [95]. It should be noted that the low success observed with DCs-based immunotherapy is due to the fact that most DCs are applied to patients in stages III and IV of the disease by a late detection of cancerous lesions, which are difficult to produce a successful immunological response with immunocompetent T lymphocytes [96, 97].

In relation to the delivery of tumor antigens for activating DCs, dead, apoptotic, or necrotic tumor cells have been used [5, 98]. DCs can phagocyte tumor cells by means of specific receptors. Thus, apoptotic cells are recognized by the integrin $\alpha V\beta 5$, by the CD36 molecule, or by means of the phosphatidylserine receptor [99] and necrotic cells are recognized by CD91, TLR-2, and TLR4 [99, 100]. One of the advantages of using dead tumor cells is that DCs can present antigens by means of MHCI activating CD8+ T lymphocytes by cross-presentation. In addition, the haplotype by which the antigens are presented is independent of the response, so this type of vaccine can be applied to any patient [3]. These types of vaccines have been shown to induce the activation of tumor-specific CD4+ and CD8+ T cells, as demonstrated by a study with 13 melanoma patients, where 3 showed tumor regression and 1 showed increased IFN levels [101].

Another strategy is the transfection of DCs with tumor RNA or encoding co-stimulatory molecules, cytokines, or growth factors [102]. DCs that have been transfected with RNA encoding tumor antigens can present tumor proteins by means of different HLA molecules, so that a large number of CD8+ T lymphocyte clones may be activated [103]. Some of the melanoma antigens used in this therapy are MAGE, gp-100, MART-1, and p53. The results have been moderately satisfactory since the development of an antitumor immune response characterized by the presence of CD8+ T lymphocytes and IFN secretion was observed; nonetheless, tumor regression was observed several times. Despite the moderate response, this type of vaccine has been shown to not only stimulate the proliferation and activation of NK cells but also induce a decrease in Treg cell levels in melanoma patients [104, 105].

Regarding the cytokines or growth factors used to activate or differentiate DCs in antitumor immunotherapy treatments, GM-CSF is one of the most widely used, since it can induce differentiation of DCs and monocytes *in vivo* [104]. On the other hand, RNA encoding for IFN, IL-7, and TNF has been transfected into DCs, resulting in cytokine secretion and DCs maturation. In some assays, it has also been attempted to transfect cells with RNA encoding cytokines, tumor antigens, and co-stimulatory molecules with the aim that with a single transfection and without the need for incubations of 24–48 h with cytokines or tumor antigens, the cells can present antigens and secrete cytokines [106].

4. Conclusions

Several aspects of the biology of DCs have been clarified, however are still missing some issues to be resolved.

1. Nonetheless in mice some precursors have been established for different subpopulations of DCs, in humans it is still necessary to clarify precisely which are the immediate precursors of the different subpopulations, in particular of the cDCs.
2. It is necessary to complete the phenotype of subpopulations of DCs in human. It is clear that as more molecules are described, in the future this will be a fulfilled task, but at the same time, it will make it more difficult to classify the DCs.
3. Protocols of *in vitro* differentiation of DCs from their precursors must be better defined. According to the latest studies, most of the results attributed to DCs are due to cellular heterogeneity, mixtures of DCs, and macrophages. In addition, it is also necessary to consider that there may be a mixture of DCs subpopulations. This issue is very important, especially when clinical trials are conducted against tumors or autoimmune diseases.
4. According to their location, DCs have several functions and this is always necessary to keep in mind, and more when it comes to understanding the particular immune responses of an organ or a tissue. Not all DCs have the same function; they can vary from organ to organ.

Acknowledgements

The authors wish to acknowledge the technical support of Biol. Beatriz Hernández-Téllez and M.C. Sara Judith Alvarez-Pérez. This work was supported by DGAPA-UNAM, PAPIIT IN218315, and IA207917.

Author details

Andrés Castell-Rodríguez*, Gabriela Piñón-Zárate, Miguel Herrera-Enríquez, Katia Jarquín-Yáñez and Iliana Medina-Solares

*Address all correspondence to: castell@unam.mx

Laboratory of Experimental Immunotherapy and Tissue Engineering, Department of Cell and Tissue Biology, Medicine School, National Autonomous University of Mexico, Mexico City, Mexico

References

[1] Merad M, Sathe P, Helft J, Miller J, Mortha A. The dendritic cell lineage: Ontogeny and function of dendritic cells and their subsets in the steady state and the inflamed setting. Annual Review of Immunology. 2013;**31**:563–604. DOI: 10.1146/annurev-immunol-020711-074950

[2] Liu K, Nussenzweig MC. Origin and development of dendritic cells. Immunological Reviews. 2010;**234(1)**:45–54. DOI: 10.1111/j.0105-2896.2009.00879.x

[3] Kurts C, Robinson BW, Knolle PA. Cross-priming in health and disease. Nature Reviews Immunology. 2010;**10(6)**:403–414. DOI: 10.1038/nri2780

[4] Palucka K, Ueno H, Fay J, Banchereau J. Dendritic cells and immunity against cancer. Journal of International Medicine. 2011;**269**:64–73. DOI: 10.1111/j.1365-2796.2010.02317.x

[5] Ullrich E, Ménard C, Flament C, Terme M, Mignot G, Bonmort M, et al. Dendritic cells and innate defense against tumor cells. Cytokine and Growth Factor Reviews. 2008;**19**:79–92. DOI: 10.1016/j.cytogfr.2007.10.009

[6] Ishikawa F, Niiro H, Iino T, Yoshida S, Saito N, Onohara S, et al. The developmental program of human dendritic cells is operated independently of conventional myeloid and lymphoid pathways. Blood. 2007;**110(10)**:3591–3660. DOI: 10.1182/blood-2007-02-071613

[7] Naik SH, Proietto AI, Wilson NS, Dakic A, Schnorrer P, Fuchsberger M, et al. Cutting edge: Generation of splenic CD8+ and CD8− dendritic cell equivalents in Fms-like tyrosine kinase 3 ligand bone marrow cultures. The Journal of Immunology. 2005;**174(11)**:6592–6597. DOI: 10.4049/jimmunol.174.11.6592

[8] Waskow C, Liu K, Darrasse-Jesé G, Guermonprez P, Ginhoux F, Merad M, et al. The receptor of tyrosine kinase Flt3 is required from dendritic cell development in peripheral lymphoid tissue. Nature Immunology. 2008;**9(9)**:676–683. DOI: 10.1038/ni.1615

[9] Warowich SS, Liu YJ. Mechanisms regulating dendritic cell specification and development. Immunology Reviews. 2010;**238**:76–92. DOI: 10.1111/j.1600-065X.2010.00949.x

[10] Purh S, Lee J, Zvezdova E, Zhou YJ, Liu K. Dendritic cell development—History, advances and open questions. Seminars in Immunology. 2015;**27**:388–396. DOI: 10.1016/j.smim.2016.03.012

[11] Bhattacharya P, Thiruppathi M, Elshabrawy HA, Alharshawi K, Kumar P, Prabhakar BS. GM-CSF: An immune modulatory cytokine that can suppress autoimmunity. Cytokine. 2015;**75**:261–271. DOI: 10.1016/j.cyto.2015.05.030

[12] Ushach I, Zlotnik A. Biological role of granulocyte macrophage colony-stimulating factor (GM-CSF) and macrophage colony-stimulating factor (M-CSF) on cells of the myeloid lineage. Journal of Leukocyte Biology. 2016;**100(3)**:481–489. DOI: 10.1189/jlb.3RU0316-144R

[13] Onai N, Obata-Onai A, Schmid MA, Ohteki T, Jarrosay D, Manz MG. Identification of clonogenic Flt3+ M-CSFR+ plasmacytoid and conventional dendritic cell progenitors in mouse bone marrow. Nature Immunology. 2007;**8(11)**:207–217. DOI: 10.1038/ni1518

[14] Fogg DK, Sibon C, Miled C, Jung S, Aucouturier P, Littman DR, et al. A clonogenic bone marrow progenitor specific for macrophages and dendritic cells. Science. 2006;**3**:83–87. DOI: 10.1126/science.1117729

[15] Naik SH, Sathe P, Park HY, Metcalf D, Proietto A, Dakic A, et al. Development of plasmacytoid and conventional dendritic cell subtypes from single precursor cells

derived in vitro and in vivo. Nature Immunology. 2007;**8(11)**:1217–1226. DOI: 10.1038/ni1522

[16] Naik SH, Perié L. Toward defining a 'lineage'—The case for dendritic cells. Seminars in Cell & Developmental Biology. 2015;**41**:3–8. DOI: 10.1016/j.semcdb.2015.02.004

[17] Guilliams M, Ginhoux F, Jakubzick C, Naik SH, Onai N, Schraml BU, et al. Dendritic cells, monocytes and macrophages: A unified nomenclature based on ontogeny. Nature Reviews Immunology. 2014;**14(8)**:571–578. DOI: 10.1038/nri3712

[18] Ginhoux F, Merad M. Ontogeny and homeostasis of Langerhans cells. Immunology & Cell Biology. 2010;**88(4)**:387–392. DOI: 10.1038/icb.2010.38

[19] Maraskovsky E, Brasel K, Teepe M, Roux ER, Lyman SD, Shortman K, et al. Dramatic increase in the numbers of functionally mature dendritic cells in Flt3ligand-treated mice: multiple dendritic cell subpopulations identified. The Journal of Experimental Medicine. 1996;**184(5)**:1953–1962. DOI: 10.1084/jem.184.5.1953

[20] Durand M, Segura E. The known unknowns of the human dendritic cell network. Frontiers in Immunology. 2015;**6**:129. DOI: 10.3389/fimmu.2015.00129

[21] Lewis KL, Caton ML, Bogunovic M, Greter M, Grajkowska LT, Ng D, et al. Notch2 receptor signaling controls functional differentiation of dendritic cells in the spleen and intestine. Immunity. 2011;**35(5)**:780–91. DOI: 10.1016/j.immuni.2011.08.013

[22] Shortman K, Liu YJ. Mouse and human dendritic cell subtypes. Nature Reviews Immunology. 2002;**2**:151–161. DOI: 10.1038/nri746

[23] Bonasio R, Scimone ML, Schaerli P, Grabie N, Lichtman AH, von Andrian UH. Clonal deletion of thymocytes by circulating dendritic cells homing to the thymus. Nature Immunology. 2006;**7**:1092–1100. DOI: 10.1038/ni1385

[24] Zhou LJ, Tedder TF. A distinct pattern of cytokine gene expression by human CD83+ blood dendritic cells. Blood. 1995;**86(9)**:3295–3301. DOI: http://www.bloodjournal.org/content/bloodjournal/86/9/3295.full.pdf

[25] Dzionek A, Fuchs A, Schmidt P, Cremer S, Zysk M, Miltenyi S, et al. BDCA-2, BDCA-3, and BDCA-4: Three markers for distinct subsets of dendritic cells in human peripheral blood. Journal of Immunology. 2000;**165(11)**:6037–6046. DOI: 10.4049/jimmunol.165.11.6037

[26] Hémont C, Neel A, Heslan M, Braudeau C, Josien R. Human blood mDC subsets exhibit distinct TLR repertoire and responsiveness. Journal of Leukocyte Biology. 2013;**93(4)**:599–609. DOI: 10.1189/jlb.0912452

[27] Bauer T, Zagorska A, Jurkin J, Yasmin N, Koffer R, Richter S, et al. Identification of axel as a downstream effector of TGF-β1 during Langerhans cells differentiation and epidermal homeostasis. The Journal of Experimental Medicine. 2012;**209(11)**:2033–2047. DOI: 10.1084/jem.20120493

[28] Seneschal J, Clark RA, Gehad A, Beacher-Allan CM, Kupper TS. Human epidermal Langerhans cells maintain immune homeostasis in skin by activating skin resident regulatory T cells. Immunity. 2012;**36**:873–884. DOI: 10.1016/j.immuni.2012.03.018

[29] De Vries IJM, Bersen MR, Lesterhuis WJ, Scharenborg NM, Strijk SP, Gerritsen MJP, et al. Immunomonitoring tumor specific T cells in delayed—type hypersensitivity skin biopsies after dendritic cell vaccination correlates with clinical outcome. Journal of Clinical Oncology. 2005;**23(24)**:5779–5787. DOI: 10.1200/JCO.2005.06.478

[30] Bogunovic M, Ginhoux F, Helft J, Shang L, Hashimoto D, Greter M, et al. Origin of the lamina propria dendritic cell network. Immunity. 2009;**31(3)**:513–525. DOI: 10.1016/j.immuni.2009.08.010

[31] De Saint-Vis B, Fugier-Vivier I, Massacrier C, Gaillard C, Vanbervliet B, Aït-Yahia S, et al. The cytokine profile expressed by human dendritic cells is dependent on cell subtype and mode of activation. Journal of Immunology. 1998;**160**:1666–1676. http://www.jimmunol.org.pbidi.unam.mx:8080/content/160/4/1666.full.pdf+html

[32] Fukao T, Matsuda S, Koyasu S. Synergistic effects of IL-4 and IL-18 on IL-12-dependent IFN-γ production by dendritic cells. Journal of Immunology. 2000;**164**:64–71. DOI: 10.4049/jimmunol.164.1.64

[33] Fanger NA, Voigtlaender D, Liu C, Swink S, Wardwell K, Fisher J, et al. Characterization of expression, cytokine regulation, and effector function of the high affinity IgG receptor Fc gamma RI (CD64) expressed on human blood dendritic cells. Journal of Immunology. 1997;**158(7)**:3090–3098. DOI: 10.4049/jimmunol.164.1.64

[34] Da Motta RJ, Tirapelli C, Juns da Silva R, Villafuerte KR, Almeida LY, Ribeiro-Silva A, et al. Immature, but not mature, dendritic cells are more often present in aggressive periodontitis than chronic periodontitis: An immunohistochemical study. Journal of Periodontology. 2016;**87(12)**:1499–1507. DOI: 10.1902/jop.2016.150729

[35] Jiang W, Swiggard WJ, Heufler C, Peng M, Mirza A, Steinman RM, et al. The receptor DEC-205 expressed by dendritic cells and thymic epithelial cells is involved in antigen processing. Nature. 1995;**375(6527)**:151–155. DOI: 10.1038/375151a0

[36] Geijtenbeek TB, Kwon DS, Torensma R, van Vliet SJ, van Duijnhoven GC, Middel J, et al. DC-SIGN, a dendritic cell-specific HIV-1-binding protein that enhances trans-infection of T cells. Cell. 2000;**100(5)**:587–597. DOI: http://dx.doi.org/10.1016/S0092-8674(00)80694-7

[37] Schreibelt G, Klinkenberg LJ, Cruz LJ, Tacken PJ, Tel J, Kreutz M, Adema GJ, et al. The C-type lectin receptor CLEC9A mediates antigen uptake and (cross-) presentation by human blood BDCA3+ myeloid dendritic cells. Blood. 2012;**119**:2284–2292. DOI: https://doi.org/10.1182/blood-2011-08-373944

[38] Fernandez NC, Lozier A, Flament C, Ricciardi-Castagnoli P, Bellet D, Suter M, et al. Dendritic cells directly trigger NK cell functions: Cross-talk relevant in innate anti-tumor immune responses in vivo. Nature Medicine. 1999;**5(4)**:405–411. DOI: 10.1038/7403

[39] Mackay F, Woodcock SA, Lawton P, Ambrose C, Baetscher M, Schneider P, et al. Mice transgenic for BAFF develop lymphocytic disorders along with autoimmune manifestations. The Journal of Experimental Medicine. 1999;**190(11)**:1697–1710. DOI: https://www-ncbi-nlm-nih-gov.pbidi.unam.mx:2443/pmc/articles/PMC2195729/

[40] Morelli AE, Zahorchak AF, Larregina AT, Colvin BL, Logar AJ, Takayama T, et al. Cytokine production by mouse myeloid dendritic cells in relation to differentiation and terminal maturation induced by lipopolysaccharide or CD40 ligation. Blood. 2001;**98**:1512–1523. DOI: 10.1182/blood.V98.5.1512

[41] Wang YS, Chi KH, Chu RM. Cytokine profiles of canine monocyte-derived dendritic cells as a function of lipopolysaccharide- or tumor necrosis factor-alpha-induced maturation. Veterinary Immunology and Immunopathology. 2007;**118**:186–198. DOI: 10.1016/j.vetimm.2007.05.010

[42] Si C, Zhang R, Wu T, Lu G, Hu Y, Zhang H, et al. Dendritic cell-derived nitric oxide inhibits the differentiation of effector dendritic cells. Oncotarget. 2016;**7(46)**:74834–74845. DOI: 10.18632/oncotarget.11361

[43] Steinbrink K, Wolfl M, Jonuleit H, Knop J, Enk AH. Induction of tolerance by IL-10-treated dendritic cells. Journal of Immunology. 1997;**159**:4772–80. DOI: http://www.jimmunol.org.pbidi.unam.mx:8080/content/159/10/4772.long

[44] Fogel-Petrovic M, Long JA, Misso NL, Foster PS, Bhoola KD, Thompson PJ. Physiological concentrations of transforming growth factor beta1 selectively inhibit human dendritic cell function. International Immunopharmacology. 2007;**7**:1924–1933. DOI: 10.1016/j.intimp.2007.07.003

[45] Hegde S, Pahne J, Smola-Hess S. Novel immunosuppressive properties of interleukin-6 in dendritic cells: Inhibition of NF-kappaB binding activity and CCR7 expression. FASEB Journal. 2004;**18**:1439–1441. DOI: 10.1096/fj.03-0969fje

[46] Menges M, Rossner S, Voigtlander C, Schindler H, Kukutsch NA, Bogdan C, et al. Repetitive injections of dendritic cells matured with tumor necrosis factor alpha induce antigen-specific protection of mice from autoimmunity. The Journal of Experimental Medicine. 2002;**195**:15–21. DOI: 10.1084/jem.20011341

[47] Garate D, Rojas-Colonelli N, Pena C, Salazar L, Abello P, Pesce B, et al. Blocking of p38 and transforming growth factor beta receptor pathways impairs the ability of tolerogenic dendritic cells to suppress murine arthritis. Arthritis Rheumatology. 2013;**65**:120–129. DOI: 10.1002/art.37702

[48] Maggi J, Schinnerling K, Pesce B, Hilkens CM, Catalán D, Aguillón JC. Dexamethasone and monophosphoryl lipid A-modulated dendritic cells promote antigen-specific tolerogenic properties on naive and memory CD4+ T cells. Frontiers in Immunology. 2016;**7**:359. DOI: 10.3389/fimmu.2016.00359

[49] Matsumoto T, Hasegawa H, Onishi S, Ishizaki J, Suemori K, Yasukawa M. Protein kinase C inhibitor generates stable human tolerogenic dendritic cells. Journal of Immunology. 2013;**191**:2247–2257. DOI: 10.4049/jimmunol.1203053

[50] Ko HJ, Cho ML, Lee SY, Oh HJ, Heo YJ, Moon YM, et al. CTLA4-Ig modifies dendritic cells from mice with collagen-induced arthritis to increase the CD4+ CD25+ Foxp3+ regulatory T cell population. Journal of Autoimmunity. 2010;**34**:111–120. DOI: 10.1016/j.jaut.2009.07.006

[51] Naranjo-Gomez M, Raich-Regue D, Onate C, Grau-Lopez L, Ramo-Tello C, Pujol-Borrell R, et al. Comparative study of clinical grade human tolerogenic dendritic cells. Journal of Translational Medicine. 2011;**9**:89. DOI: 10.1186/1479-5876-9-89

[52] Kryczanowsky F, Raker V, Graulich E, Domogalla MP, Steinbrink K. IL-10-modulated human dendritic cells for clinical use: Identification of a stable and migratory subset with improved tolerogenic activity. Journal of Immunology. 2016;**197**:3607–3617. DOI: 10.4049/jimmunol.1501769

[53] Roelen DL, van den Boogaardt DE, van Miert PP, Koekkoek K, Offringa R, Claas FH. Differentially modulated dendritic cells induce regulatory T cells with different characteristics. Transplant Immunology. 2008;**19(3–4)**:220–228. DOI: 10.1016/j.trim.2008.06.004

[54] Cisse B, Caton ML, Lehner M, Maeda T, Scheu S, Locksley R, et al. Transcription factor E2-2 is an essential and specific regulator of plasmacytoid dendritic cell development. Cell. 2008;**135**:37–48. DOI: 10.1016/j.cell.2008.09.016

[55] Ghosh HS, Cisse B, Bunin A, Lewis KL, Reizis B. Continuous expression of the transcription factor E2-2 maintains the cell fate of mature plasmacytoid dendritic cells. Immunity. 2010;**33(6)**:905–916. DOI: 10.1016/j.immuni.2010.11.023

[56] Villadangos JA, Young L. Antigen-presentation properties of plasmacytoid dendritic cells. Immunity. 2008;**29**:352–361. DOI: 10.1016/j.immuni.2008.09.002

[57] Reizis B, Colonna M, Trinchieri G, Barrat F and Gilliet M. Plasmacytoid dendritic cells: One-trick ponies or workhorses of the immune system? Nature Reviews Immunology. 2011;**11**:558–565. DOI: 10.1038/nri3027

[58] Fallarino F, Asselin-Paturel C, Vacca C, Bianchi R, Gizzi S, Fioretti MC, et al. Murine plasmacytoid dendritic cells initiate the immunosuppressive pathway of tryptophan catabolism in response to CD200 receptor engagement. Journal of Immunology. 2004;**173(6)**:3748–3754. DOI: https://doi.org/10.4049/jimmunol.173.6.3748

[59] Klechevsky E, Flamar AL, Cao Y, Blanck JP, Liu M, O'Bar A, et al. Cross-priming CD8 T cells by targeting antigens to human dendritic cells through DCIR. Current Opinion in Immunology. 2006;**8(1)**:85–91. DOI: 10.1182/blood-2010-01-264960

[60] Joffre OP, Segura E, Savina A, Amigorena S. Cross-presentation by dendritic cells. Nature Reviews Immunology. 2012;**12(8)**:557–569. DOI: 10.1038/nri3254

[61] Madden DR. The three-dimensional structure of peptide-MHC complexes. Annual Review of Immunology. 1995;**13**:587. DOI: 10.1146/annurev.iy.13.040195.003103

[62] Chapman HA. Endosomal proteases in antigen presentation. Current Opinion in Immunology. 2006;**18**:78–84. DOI: 10.1016/j.coi.2005.11.011

[63] Ackerman AL, Cresswell P. Cellular mechanisms governing cross-presentation of exogenous antigens. Nature Immunology. 2004;**5**:678. DOI: 10.1038/ni1082

[64] Guermonprez P, Amigorena S. Pathways for antigen cross presentation. Springer Seminars in Immunopathology. 2005;**26**:257–271. DOI: 10.1007/s00281-004-0176-0

[65] Basta S, Alatery A. The cross-priming pathway: A portrait of an intricate immune system. Scandinavian Journal of Immunology. 2007;**65**:311–319. DOI: 10.1111/j.1365-3083.2007.01909.x

[66] Shen L, Rock KL. Priming of T cells by exogenous antigen cross-presented on MHC class I molecules. Current Opinion in Immunology. 2006;**18**:85–91. DOI 10.1016/j.coi.2005.11.003

[67] Rock KL, York IA, Goldberg. AL.Post-proteosomal antigen processing for major histocompatibility complex class I presentation. Nature Immunology. 2004;**5**:670. DOI: 10.1038/ni1089

[68] Klechevsky E. Functional diversity of human dendritic cells. Advances in Experimental Medicine and Biology. 2015;**850**:43–54. DOI: 10.1007/978-3-319-15774-0_4

[69] Gutiérrez-Martínez E, Planès R, Anselmi G, Reynolds M, Menezes S, Adiko AC, et al. Cross presentation of cell-associated antigens by MHC class I in dendritic cell subsets. Frontiers in Immunology. 2015;**6**:363. DOI: 10.3389/fimmu.2015.00363

[70] BrodeS,MacaryPA.Cross-presentation:Dendriticcellsandmacrophagesbiteoffmorethan they can chew! Immunology. 2004;**112(3)**:345–351. DOI: 10.1111/j.1365-2567.2004.01920.x

[71] Yazdi S, Röcken M, Ghoreschi K. Cutaneous immunology: Basics and new concepts. Seminar in Immunopathology. 2016;**38**:3–10. DOI 10.1007/s00281-015-0545-x

[72] Honda T, Egawa G, Grabbe S, Kabashima K. Update of immune events in the murine contact hypersensitivity model: Toward the understanding of allergic contact dermatitis. Journal of Investigative Dermatology. 2013;**133(2)**:303–315. DOI: 10.1038/jid.2012.284 103

[73] Biedermann T, Kneilling M, Mailhammer R et al. Mast cells control neutrophil recruitment during T cell mediated delayed-type hypersensitivity reactions through tumor necrosis factor and macrophage inflammatory protein 2. The Journal of Experimental Medicine. 2000;**192**:1441–1451. DOI: http://www.jem.org/cgi/content/full/192/10/1441

[74] Clausen BE, Stoitzner P. Functional specialization of skin dendritic cell subsets in regulating T cell responses. Frontiers in Immunology. 2015;**6**:534. DOI: 10.3389/fimmu.2015.00534

[75] Kaplan DH, Igyártó BZ, Gaspari AA. Early immune events in the induction of allergic contact dermatitis. Nature Reviews Immunology. 2012;**12(2)**:114–124. DOI: 10.1038/nri3150

[76] Biedermann T1, Mailhammer R, Mai A, Sander C, Ogilvie A, Brombacher F, et al. Reversal of established delayed type hypersensitivity reactions following therapy with IL-4 or antigen-specific Th2 cells. European Journal of Immunology. 2001;**31**:1582–1591. DOI: 10.1002/1521-4141(200105)31:5<1582::AID-IMMU1582>3.0.CO;2-M

[77] Banchereau J, Steinman R. Dendritic cells and the control of immunity. Nature. 1998;**392**:245–252. DOI: 10.1038/32588

[78] Ohnmacht C, Pulver A, Hing S, Drexler I, Meier S, Brocken T, et al. Constitutive ablation of dendritic cells breaks self-tolerance of CD4 T cells and results in spontaneous fatal autoimmunity. The Journal of Experimental Medicine. 2009;**206(3)**:549–559. DOI: 10.1084/jem.20082394

[79] Paterka M, Voss JO, Werr J, Reuter E, Franck S, Leuenberger T, et al. Dendritic cells tip the balance towards induction of regulatory T cells upon priming in experimentalautoimmune encephalomyelitis. Journal of Autoimmunity. 2016;**76**:108–114. DOI: 10.1016/j.jaut.2016.09.008

[80] Mahnke YD, Brodie TM, Sallusto F, Roederer M, Lugli E. The who's who of T-cell differentiation: Human memory T-cell subsets. European Journal of Immunology. 2013;**43(11)**:2797–2809. DOI: 10.1002/eji.201343751

[81] Desnues B, Macedo AB, Ordoñez-Rueda D, Roussel-Queval A, Malissen B, Bruhns P, et al. The transcriptional repressor Gfi1 prevents lupus autoimmunity by restraining TLR7 signaling. European Journal of Immunology. 2016;**46(12)**:2801–2811. DOI: 10.1002/eji.201646573

[82] Greter M, Heppner FL, Lemos MP, Odermatt BM, Goebels N, Laufer N. Dendritic cells permit immune invasion of the CNS in an animal model of multiple sclerosis. Nature Medicine. 2005;**11**:328–334. DOI: 10.1038/nm1197

[83] Chalise JP, Pallotta MT, Chenna Narendra S, Carlsson B, Iacono A, Namale J, et al. IDO1 and TGF-1 β mediate protective effects of IFN-αin antigen-induced arthritis. Journal of Immunology. 2016;**197(8)**:3142–3151. DOI: 10.4049/jimmunol.1502125

[84] Hanahan D, Weinberg RA. Hallmarks of cancer: The next generation. Cell. 2011;**144(5)**: 646–674. DOI: dx.doi.org/10.1016/j.cell.2011.02.013

[85] Fridman WH, Pagès F, Sautès-Fridman C, Galon J. The immune contexture in human tumours: Impact on clinical outcome. Nature Reviews Cancer. 2012;**12(4)**:298–306. DOI: 10.1038/nrc3245

[86] Enk A, Jonuleit H, Saloga J, Knop J. Dendritic cells as mediators of tumor induced tolerance in metastatic melanoma. International Journal of Cancer. 1997;**73**:309–316. DOI: 10.1002/(SICI)1097-0215(19971104)73:3<309::AID-IJC1>3.0.CO;2-3

[87] Scarlett UK, Rutkowski MR, Rauwerdink AM, Fields J, Escovar-Fadul X, Baird J, et al. Ovarian cancer progression is controlled by phenotypic changes in dendritic cells. The Journal of Experimental Medicine. 2012;**209(3)**:495–506. DOI: 10.1084/jem.20111413

[88] Stagg J, Johnstone R, Smyth M. From cancer immunosurveillance to cancer immunotherapy. Immunological Reviews. 2007;**220**:82–101. DOI: 10.1111/j.1600-065X.2007.00566.x

[89] Bhardwaj N, Gnjatic S, Sawhney NB. TLR agonists: Are they good adjuvants? Cancer Journal. 2010;**16(4)**:382–391. DOI: 10.1097/PPO.0b013e3181eaca65

[90] Zytvogel L, Apetoh L, Ghiringhelli F, Kroemer G. Immunological aspects of cancer chemotherapy. Nature Reviews of Immunology. 2008;**8**:59–73. DOI: 10.1038/nri2216

[91] Zhang Y, Sun Z, Nicolay H, Meyer RG, Renkvist N, Stroobant V. Monitoring of anti-vaccine CD4 T cell frequencies in melanoma patients vaccinated with MAGE-3 protein. Journal of Immunology. 2005;**174**:2404–2411. DOI: https://doi.org/10.4049/jimmunol.174.4.2404

[92] Carrasco J, Van Pel A, Neys B, Lethé B, Brasseur F, Renkvist N, et al. Vaccination of a melanoma patient with mature dendritic cells pulsed with MAGE-3 peptides triggers the activity of nonvaccine anti-tumor cells. Journal of Immunology. 2008;**180**:3585–3593. DOI: https://doi.org/10.4049/jimmunol.180.5.3585

[93] Grover A, Kim GJ, Lizée G, Tschoi M, Wang G, Wunderlich JR et al. Intralymphatic dendritic cell vaccination induces tumor antigen– specific, skin-homing T lymphocytes. Clinical Cancer Research. 2006;**12**:5801–5808. DOI: 10.1158/1078-0432.CCR-05-2421

[94] Slingluff CL, Petroni CR, Yamshchikov GV, Barnd DL, Eastham S, Galavotti H, et al. Clinical and immunologic results of a randomized phase II trial of vaccination using four melanoma peptides either administered in granulocyte-macrophage colony-stimulating factor in adjuvant or pulsed on dendritic cells. Journal of Clinical Oncology. 2003;**21**:4016–4026. DOI: 10.1200/JCO.2003.10.005

[95] Lonchay C, Van der Bruggen, Cannerotte T, Hanagiri T, Coulie P, Colau D, et al. Correlation between tumor regression and T cell responses in melanoma patients vaccinated with a MAGE antigen. PNAS. 2004;**101**:14631–14638. DOI: 10.1073/pnas.0405 743101

[96] Xia D, Moyana T, Xiang J. Combinational adenovirus-mediated gene therapy and dendritic cell vaccine in combating well-established tumors. Journal of Cell Research. 2006;**16**:241–259. DOI: 10.1038/sj.cr.7310032

[97] Lubaroff DM, Karan D. CpG oligonucleotide as an adjuvant for the treatment of prostate cancer. Advanced Drug Delivery Reviews. 2009;**61**:268–274. DOI: 10.1016/j.addr.2008.12.005

[98] Fields RC, Shimizu K, Mule JJ. Murine dendritic cells pulsed with whole tumor lysates mediate potent antitumor immune responses in vitro and in vivo. Proceedings of the National Academy of Science USA. 1998;**95**:9482–9487. DOI: https://www-ncbi-nlm-nih-gov.pbidi.unam.mx:2443/pmc/articles/PMC21364/

[99] Dhodapkar MV, Dhodapkar KM, Palucka AK. Interactions of tumor cells with dendritic cells: Balancing immunity and tolerance. Cell Death and Differentiation. 2008;**15**:39–50. DOI: 10.1038/sj.cdd.4402247

[100] Apetoh L, Ghringheli F, Tesnieres A, Obeid M, Ortiz C, Criollo A, et al. Toll like receptor 4 dependent contribution of the immune system to anticancer chemotherapy and radiotherapy. Nature Medicine. 2004;**13**:1051–1060. DOI: 10.1038/nm1622

[101] Palucka AK, Ueno H, Connolly J, Kerneis-Norvell F, Blanck JP, Johnston DA, et al. Dendritic cells loaded with killed allogeneic melanoma cells can induce objective clinical responses and MART-1 specific CD8+ T-cell immunity. Journal of Immunotherapy. 2006;**29**:545–557. DOI: 10.1097/01.cji.0000211309.90621.8b

[102] Ribas A, Butterfield LH, William H. McBride WH, Dissette VB, Koh A, et al. Characterization of antitumor immunization to a defined melanoma antigen using genetically engineered murine dendritic cells. Cancer Gene Therapy. 1999;**6**:523–536. DOI: 10.1038/sj.cgt.7700076

[103] Boczkowski D, Nair SK, Nam JH, Lyerly HK, Gilboa E. Induction of tumor immunity and cytotoxic T lymphocyte responses using dendritic cells transfected with messenger RNA amplified from tumor cells. Cancer Research. 2000;**60**:1028–1034. DOI: http://cancerres.aacrjournals.org.pbidi.unam.mx:8080/content/canres/60/4/1028.full.pdf

[104] Liu Y, Santin AD, Mane M, Chiriva-Internati M, Parham GP, Ravaggi A, et al. Transduction and utility of the granulocyte-macrophage colony-stimulating factor gene into monocytes and dendritic cells by adeno-associated virus. Journal of Interferon Cytokine Research. 2000;**20**:21–30. DOI: 10.1089/107999000312702

[105] Bray SM, Vujanovic L, Butterfield LH. Dendritic cell-based vaccines positively impact natural killer and regulatory T cells in hepatocellular carcinoma patients. Clinical and Developmental Immunology. 2011;**2011**:1–11. DOI: 10.1155/2011/249281

[106] Sheng KC, Pietersz GA, Wright M. Apostolopoulos V. Dendritic cells: Activation and maturation, application for cancer immunotherapy. Current Medicinal Chemistry. 2005;**12**:1783–1800. DOI: https://doi.org/10.2174/0929867054367248

[107] Li MO, Wan YY, Sanjabi S, Robertson AKL, Flavell RA. Transforming Growth Factor-β regulation of immune response. Annu Rev Immunol. 2006;**24**:99-146. DOI:10.1146/annurev.immunol.24.021605.090737

Section 2

Function in Organ and Disease

Chapter 3

The Biological Function of Kupffer Cells in Liver Disease

Yuan-yuan Ma, Mu-qing Yang, Zhi-gang He,
Qing Wei and Ji-yu Li

Additional information is available at the end of the chapter

http://dx.doi.org/10.5772/67673

Abstract

Kupffer cells, which have a characteristic morphology and a kind of phenotype, are the resident macrophages in liver, serve as the largest population mononuclear phagocytes in the body, and are localized in the periportal zone. They have phagocytosis capacity and release all kinds of cytokines, chemokines, and soluble biological mediators. Owing to the different functions of Kupffer cells, they play an important role in liver diseases. In this chapter, we review the role of Kupffer cells in infectious disease, fatty liver disease, liver fibrosis, liver ischemia-reperfusion injury, liver transplantation immunology, as well as liver cancer and metastases.

Keywords: Kupffer cell, infectious disease, fatty liver disease, fibrosis, ischemia-reperfusion injury, liver transplantation immunology, liver cancer, metastases

1. Introduction

Kupffer cells (KCs), as the largest population mononuclear phagocytes in the body, account for 80–90% of the total number of natural macrophages and 20% of the liver nonparenchymal cells [1]. They form a self-renewing pool of organ-resident macrophages independent of the myeloid monocyte compartment and derive from resident stem cells which originate from the fetal yolk sac before [2–4]. Other studies also found that KCs derived from embryonic progenitors colonize the tissues before birth [5–11], but with the growth of mouse, bone marrow-derived monocytes will fill up additional macrophage niches that become available, competing with the resident population. This situation occurs in the liver and spleen, but not in the brain and lung [12].

KCs have a characteristic morphology with amoeboid lamellipodia and an irregular surface containing many microvilli [13], located at the luminal side of liver sinusoidal endothelium or the lamellipodia extended into the Disse space through the fenestrae. This is an ideal position for their main function in the liver. This state can filter the blood that enters the liver from both the portal vein and the hepatic artery, which is an important part of the cellular immunity system of the mammalia (**Figure 1**). So, the structure of KCs plays a role in the mutual coordination and influence of liver parenchymal cells and other nonparenchymal cell functions and makes up these cells' important versatile constituents of the liver [14–16]. Now, according to the function of KCs, they could be distinguished as two groups: the one with higher phagocytosis capacity and the other with preference toward cytokines and chemokines production [17, 18]. Some studies found that there were large KCs in rats. They are localized in the periportal zone and have increased phagocytosis and increased production of biological mediators. These large KCs can be identified by the expression of CD163, also described as ED2 antigen, which is a scavenger receptor [19]. KCs (**Table 1**) can also be identified by the expression of CD68 (ED-1); they were called small KCs in rats. The general macrophage marker F4/80 or by ED-1 was expressed on the surface of mice KCs, which is present in all KCs regardless of their location [20]. In mice, KCs can be distinguished from monocytes among the F4/80$^+$ cells as Ly6C low CD11b low-cell population [21, 22]. Additionally, macrophages are functionally grouped into two classes, M1 and M2. M1 (termed classically activated) macrophages are pro-inflammatory and could produce pro-inflammatory cytokines and chemokines, while the M2 (termed alternatively activated) macrophages are suppressive and involved in cellular repair [23]. According to this situation, KCs as one kind of macrophages also have these functions and play a fundamental role in homeostasis and diseases [24]. KCs also have a unique KCs gene Clec4f to distinguish with other macrophage; Clec4F has been previously described as a KCs-specific marker [25–27].

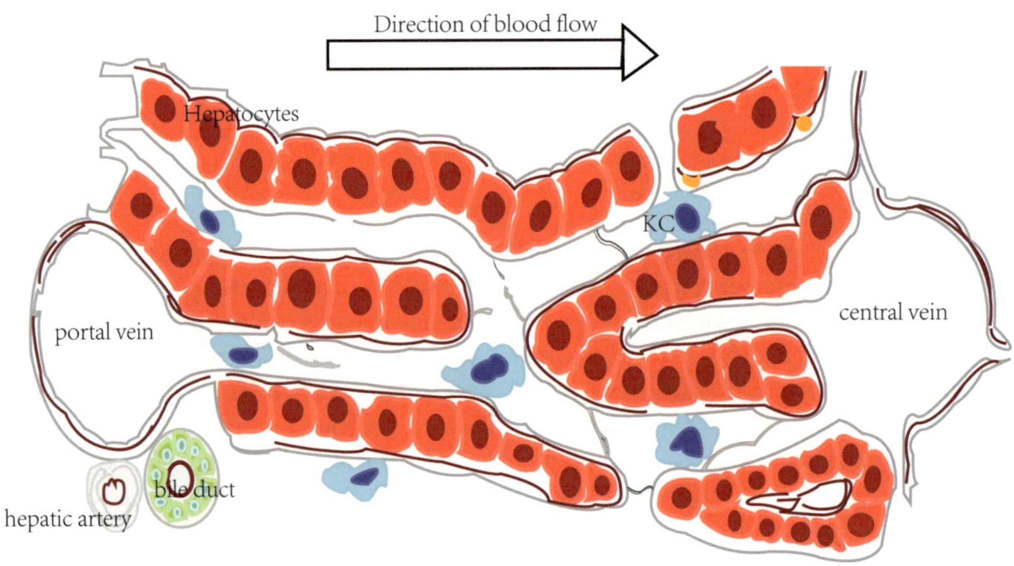

Figure 1. Schematic representation of the liver microanatomical structure and Kupffer cell localization in lower magnification.

	Origin	Marker	PRR	PAMP DAMP	Immunogenic	Polarization of macrophages	
Rat	Derived from the fetal yolk sack and embryonic progenitors colonize the tissues. Liver-resident Express Clec4F gene	CD68/ED1 CD163/ED2	Scavengers receptors (CDl3, CD14, CDl5, CD68, CD163) Mannose receptors Fc receptors (CD64, CD32, CDl6) Complement receptor (CR1, CR3, CR4) I region-associated antigen	TLR1-TLR9 NLR	MHC-II CD80 CD86 PDL-1 (CD274)	M1	Pro-inflammatory antitumoral
Mouse		F4/80 CD68 $CD11b^{low}$		TLR1-TLR9 NLR RLR		M2	Anti-inflammatory Immune suppressive protumoral
Human		CD68 CD14		TLR2 TLR3 TLR4 NLR			

Table 1. This table is used for KC identification and major surface receptors and moleculars involved in the function in human, mouse, and rat.

In vivo, under steady condition, the KCs are resting situation; they play a role in eliminating macromolecules, immune complexes, toxins, and degenerated cells from circulation. Pattern recognition receptors (PRRs) on the KCs are the main factor to eliminate the debris, toxins, and insoluble macromolecules, such as scavengers receptors (CDl3, CD14, CDl5, and CD68, CD163), mannose receptors, Fc receptors (including CD64, CD32, and CDl6), complement receptor (including the complement receptor L, complement receptor 3, and complement receptor 4), I region-associated antigen, which are able to bind to toxins lipopolysaccharide (LPS), immune complexes, or opsonized cells [28]. Since KCs reside in the liver sinusoids in large numbers and are adherent to the endothelial cells, they are able to sample the blood entering the liver from the gut as well as from the main circulation. KCs also could remove the senescent or damaged erythrocytes. In this process, following phagocytosis and hemolysis, KCs could express HO (including HO-1, HO-2, and HO-3) to degrade hemoglobin, which is part of erythrocytes component. HO-1 catalyzes the degradation of heme into iron, biliverdin, and carbon monoxide, which are all considered to be hepatoprotective at low quantities under steady-state conditions [29, 30].

Pathogen- and damage-associated molecular patterns (PAMPs and DAMPs, respectively) were two kinds of PRRs to express on the surface of KCs. They included multiple families, such as Toll-like, RIG-like, and NOD-like receptors (TLR, RLR, and NLR, respectively), and C-type lectin receptors (CLR) [31]. Mouse KCs can express TLR1-TLR9, all of which appear to be functional [32]. Human KCs, so far, have only been described to express TLR2, TLR3, and TLR4 [33, 34]. Furthermore, in the *Listeria monocytogenes* (Lm) infection model, mouse KCs are shown to express RIG-like receptor I [35]. Hepatocytes and $CD68^+$ liver mononuclear cells (presumably KCs) express NLRC2 (NOD2) [36]. When the KCs were activated by the emergence of endotoxins and harmful exogenous particles from the portal vein and circulation, their functions were enhanced. They could produce all kinds of cytokines and chemokines significantly. In the presence of TLR ligands, such as LPS and CpG, the CD14-positive KCs were stimulated by TLR4, which activates the intracellular signal pathway via myeloid differentiation factor 88 (MyD 88), resulting in NF-κB activation to produce the pro-inflammation cytokines IL-6, TNF-α, IL-1β, ICAM-1, VCAM-1, and VAP-1 [37], and the CD14 expression on KCs is increased [31]. CD14-transgenic mice that overexpress CD14 on monocytes have increased sensitivity to LPS [38]. As a receptor of dsRNA, TLR3 on KCs is one of the primary triggers in the defense of viral diseases. TLR3 activation induces the strongest IFN-γ response. KCs were activated presumably due to the induction of IL-12 in the absence of IL-10 coproduction, which was observed upon TLR2 and TLR4 ligation [39]. Activation of TLR7 triggers the secretion of type I interferons and activation of subsequent genes encoding CXCL10, CXCL11, Mx1 (antiviral G-Protein), CCL2 (also known as MCP-1), also secretion of IL-10, leading to enhanced viral clearance [40]. TLR9 activation on KCs attenuates inflammation by the secretion of IL-10, suppressing the activation of infiltrating monocyte-derived macrophages in mice. This finding supports a dual role of TLR9 engagement, which depends on the target T-cell type [41]. LPS, DNA, SFA, amyloid cholesterol, cathepsin κ, and reactive oxygen species (ROS) and so on have been suggested as NLPR3 activators, which comprise the NOD-like receptor NLRP3, the apoptosis-associated speck-like protein containing a caspase recruitment domain, and the effector molecule procaspase inflammation [42].

KCs likely derived from infiltrating monocytes express MHC-II antigens and costimulatory molecules (CD80 and CD86), which can present foreign antigens to the reactive T cells, induced T cell responses, and thus conferred tolerance to induce regulatory T cells in immune response [28]. IL-10 and PDL-1 (also known as CD274) participated in the immune tolerance, which reduce the antigen-presenting capacity of KCs by downregulating the expression of MHC molecules and costimulators, but without strongly affecting the scavenger function of KCs.

KCs not only can interact with T cells but can also interact with many cellular components in the liver. For instance, KCs can initiate the recruitment of other monocytes to the liver in case of injuries, which is important for liver regeneration, and they also interact with hepatic stellate cells (HSCs) to play a role in liver diseases and repair [43, 44]. TLR4 signal on KCs indirectly silences patrolling NK cells by MYD88-dependent IL-10 secretion, whereas TLR2 or TLR3 induces IL-18 and IL-1β, leading to NK-cell activation in liver inflammation [45]. Traditionally, M1 macrophage phenotype is marked by the release of pro-inflammatory cytokines like TNF-κ, IL-1, and IL-12. Alternative activation of M2 phenotype is more heterogeneous, as different stimuli are main to release anti-inflammation cytokines (such as IL-10). Typically, the increased expression of arginase 1, the secretion of immune-modulatory cytokines (such as IL-10 and TGF-κ), and the involvement in tissue repair phase are considered as indicators of M2 macrophage differentiation. Different origin of the cells together with the functional plasticity of macrophages can explain the phenotypic and functional heterogeneity of KCs observed upon different triggers of liver pathology [46, 47]. On the basis of these concepts, in the next sections, we summarize the role of KCs to various diseases involving the liver, in particular infectious disease, fatty liver disease, liver fibrosis and cirrhosis, ischemia and reperfusion (I/R) injury, liver cancer as well as liver transplantation immunology (**Figure 2**).

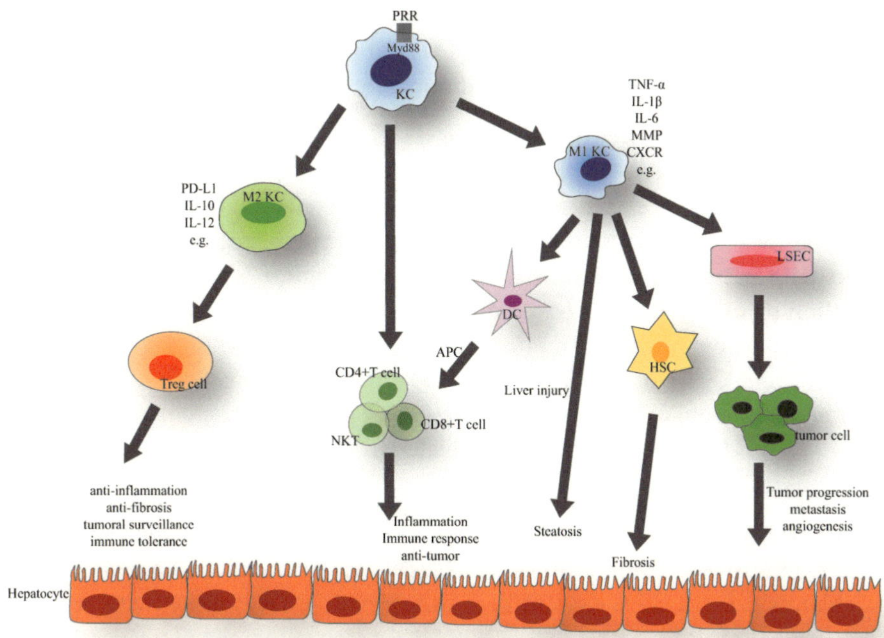

Figure 2. KCs interact with other cells in liver diseases and have the bidirectional function.

2. Kupffer cells in infectious disease

KCs and the sinusoidal endothelial cells are the first barriers for pathogens to enter the liver via the portal vein [48]. Their endocytic capacity, the expression of different PRRs, MHC, and costimulatory molecules, and the ability to produce a variety of physiologically active substances (mediators of the inflammatory process) when they were stimulated make them as the potent immune cells that aim to either pathogen clearance or persistence. The liver is constantly exposed to non–self-protein which is derived from nutrients or microbiota, and bacterial endotoxins would trigger immune response to induce inflammation. These pathogens may activate KCs that lead to produce anti-inflammation cytokines and chemokines for the inhibition of pathogen replication, or recruit and activate other immune cells to liver to participate in the inflammation reaction. So the inflammation process is a multifactor and multicell interaction to participate in. In this process, KCs can recruit other immune cells such as monocytes into the liver, which are then polarized into regulatory IL-10^{+}IL-12^{-}DCs by hepatocyte growth factor [49], macrophage colony-stimulating factor (M-CSF) [50], through inducing activation of the signal of STAT3 and SMAD, then blocking NF-κB [51], and then producing anti-inflammation cytokines. At the same time, stimulation of the body-wide DCs response by the administration of Fms-related tyrosine kinase 3 ligand (Flt3L), granulocyte colony-stimulating factor (G-CSF), or granulocyte-macrophage colony-stimulating factor (GM-CSF) reverses endotoxin-related immunoparalysis that probably over produces unprimed myeloid cells, which in turn are capable of developing into TNF-IL-12-DCs after stimulation with LPS and other pathogens [52]. This approach may effect on patients with acute-on-chronic liver failure to overcome immunoparalysis [53].

NK cells are important during liver inflammation, TLR2 or TLR3 signal on KCs are activated to induce cytokines IL-18 and IL-1β production, then lead to NK cells activation to immune responses [54]. The chemokine CXCL16 secretion from KCs could guide the CXCR6⁺ NKT-cell trafficking in the liver to regulate immune responses during microbial infection, and KCs might interact with patrolling NKT cells via glycolipid receptors such as CD1d to produce pro-inflammation cytokines IL-4, IFN-γ, and then provide cytotoxic activity [55–57]. When KCs were activated, they become immunogenic to induce CD8 T cells activation, and the generation of efficient CLT response [58, 59]. Thus, during liver infection, KCs support the development of antimicrobial T cell responses. Besides CD8 T cells responses, recent studies describe that naive CD4 T cells also could be activated in the murine liver disease [60].

The interaction of KCs with membrane-bound as well as soluble mediators expressed by infiltrating immune cells probably leads to further regulation of KCs function. Several studies have reported the involvement of adhesion molecule vascular endothelial growth factor-1 (VEGF-1), which is expressed by KCs, in liver inflammation. In common with endothelial cells which express both VCAM-1 and VEGF-Rs, KCs also could express several antigens that functionally regulate the bioactivities of KCs, including cytokine activation and production, cytoskeleton rearrangement, survival, and chemotaxis in liver inflammation [61–68]. The infiltration of neutrophils is commonly seen in all types of liver disease, especially in liver inflammation [69]. Neutrophils also could activate KCs and endothelial cells, leading to upregulation of cellular adhesion molecules such as ICAM-1, VCAM-1, or VAP-1 to induce neutrophils infiltration and endocytose the microbe [70]. Furthermore, KCs might play a dual effect in liver inflammation, and pathogens may exploit the tolerogenic capacities of KCs to evade immunity and may have evolved to inhibit the immunogenic functions of KCs. Then, we provide examples of the various roles of KCs in bacterial, viral, and parasitic infection.

2.1. Liver infection by bacteria

Kupffer cells act as sentinels capturing antigens and pathogens and are key contributors of host defense against enteroinvasive bacteria [5]. *L. monocytogenes* (Lm) is a very well-characterized facultative intracellular model microorganism [71]. Lm, which could be captured by KCs, triggers a massive recruitment of monocytes leading to the formation of liver Lm-containing microabscesses 2–3 days post inoculation [72]. These microabscesses contain M1 macrophages, TNF/iNOS-producing dendritic cells (Tip-DCs), and neutrophils to play a critical role in the rapid control of the infection [73, 74]. Infected KCs secrete inflammation mediators such as IL-1β and IL-4 to inhibit proliferation of the microorganism [75]. At the same time, infected KCs could secret chemokines such as MIP-1α (CCL3), MIP-1β (CCL4), MCP-1 (CCL2), and MIP-2 (CXCL2/-3), leading to "pro-inflammatory" M1 macrophages that express the chemokine receptor CCR2 recruitment to the liver, which egress from the bone marrow, then control the infection [76, 77]. But some studies indicate that KCs undergo a rapid necroptotic death upon the first hours of their infection by Lm. KCs necroptosis triggers hepatocytes to release the alarmin interleukin-33 (IL-33), which triggers basophil IL-4 production [78], then in turn causes recruited monocyte-derived macrophages to proliferate and shift from an M1 to M2 phenotype. This allows ultimately the replacement of dead KCs by M2 macrophages after Lm infection. During infection with Lm, tissue-resident KCs are quantitatively replaced by monocytes, which develop into tissue-resident macrophages. The lethal irradiation also led to the replacement of embryo-derived KCs by bone-marrow-derived macrophages, which acquired a highly similar cell identity as indicated by the adoption of a KCs characteristic global enhancer landscape. Initially, these cells contribute to antibacterial immunity in a typical IFN-γ-driven inflammatory response. In the second phase, KCs necroptosis also initiates a cascade of IL-4-driven events inducing proliferative expansion and phenotypic changes of monocyte-derived macrophages that promote restoration of tissue integrity after bacterial clearance. Similar results were obtained with the enteroinvasive bacterium of *Salmonella enterica* [79]. This is a new field of investigations for infection control and tissue return to homeostasis.

When liver infection with *Francisella tularensis* occurs, it is able to infect and replicate within Kupffer cells which release pro-inflammatory cytokines TNFα, IL-1β, and IL-6, leading to sepsis [80]. But hepatocytes as well as dendritic cells may support the intracellular replication of *F. tularensis* without undergoing proptosis or apoptosis, because the hepatocytes could release chemokines FKN to reverse this process [81, 82]. So, KCs inactivation or depletion results in impaired bacterial clearance. Although KCs play a critical role in infection, various studies indicate that the actual elimination of the bacteria taken up by the liver depends on a complex interaction of KC and other inflammation cells.

2.2. Liver infection by viruses

Both hepatitis B virus (HBV) and hepatitis C virus (HCV) are blood-borne viruses, when infected by them can result in chronic liver disease with an increased risk for liver fibrosis/cirrhosis, hepatic failure, and liver cancer [83, 84]. Studies suggested that hepatic macrophages played an important role in viral hepatitis. KCs have a beneficial antiviral effect on the early phase after infection. During systemic viral infection, liver resident KCs are essential for the efficient capture of the virus and preventing viral replication. The next involves fast induction of an antiviral status in KCs by producing IFN-γ and prevents viral spread to neighboring hepatocytes [85, 86]. Activated KCs express high levels of immunogenic MHC II and can thereby activate virus-specific $CD4^+$ T cells in liver; $CD4^+$ T cells also can produce IFN-γ in response to antigen exposure. At the same time, under an antiviral status, this might enhance the phagocytic capacity of KCs, which might additionally contribute to control virus replication [87, 88]. Some studies make use of a short-term LCMV-Cl13 infection in mice to examine phenotypic and functional changes in inflammatory monocytes and F4/80-high-Kupffer cells instead of virus infection animal models; these cells are the first innate immune cells to encounter a viral pathogen in liver. They observed F4/80-high-Kupffer cells, which maintain their endocytic activity and increase the expression of several pro- and anti-inflammatory cytokines and chemokines after LCMV infection. KCs from LCMV-infected mice clearly show the induction of pro- and anti-inflammatory cytokines and chemokines, including TNF, IL-6, IL-10, MCP, CXCL-10, and others. The active uptake of LCMV by KCs limits viral spread and immunopathology [89, 90].

In human body, when they are infected by HBV particles and HBs, the virus induces IL-1β, IL-6, IL-18, CXCL8, and TNF production by human CD68⁺ KCs via NF-κB activation leading to NK cell activity and then NK cells produce IFN-γ, which plays an important role in antiviral immunity.

KCs have two functional AIM2 and NLRP3 inflammasomes, and that AIM2 production of IL-1β and IL-18 is essential for IL-8 transcription as well as activating liver and peripheral blood NK cells, respectively [91, 92]. Some studies demonstrated that rat $ED1^+$-adherent KCs exposed to HBV virus hardly expressed IL-1β, IL-6, or TNF, but produced the immunoregulatory cytokine TGF-β, because hepatitis B surface Ag blocks IRF7 binding to the AIM2 promoter. Targeting AIM2 prevents the recognition of dsDNA expressed by the HBV, and that the limited innate response observed upon HBV infection may be due to viral-mediated immune evasion [93, 94]. Another link between hepatic inflammation and disease in patients with chronic HCV was attributed to IL-1β secretion following the activation of the NLRP3 inflammasome in liver macrophages ($CD68^+/CD14^+$) [95].

Chronic infection associated with hepatitis B virus (HBV) is a major cause of liver fibrosis and cirrhosis. The activation of NADPH oxidase during the phagocytosis of HBV particles, and signal transducers and activators of transcription-3 (STAT-3) binding to elements in the TGF-β promoter may also be involved to increase TGF-β production. So KCs could produce the pro-fibrogenic/anti-inflammatory cytokine TGF-β rather than the pro-inflammatory cytokines IL-6, IL-1, and TNF-α. This may partly explain why overt liver fibrosis is still present when chronic hepatitis B virus infection occurs with minimal (or no) necroinflammation [93, 96, 97]. KCs in the HBs-Tg mice expressed higher level of CD205 and produced greater amounts of interleukin (IL)-12 than did those in the WT mice. Depletion of KCs, neutralization of IL-12, or specific silencing of CD205 on KCs significantly inhibited CpG-oligodeoxynucleotides (CpG-ODN)-induced liver injury and NKT cells activation in the HBs-Tg mice. These data CD205-expressing KCs respond to CpG-ODNs and subsequently release IL-12 to promote NKT cell activation. Activated NKT cells induce liver damage through the Fas-signaling pathway in HBs-Tg mice [98].

HCV infection also could make KCs and liver-infiltrating lymphocytes the major sources of TGF-protein, leading to liver fibrosis [99]. The cellular protein, glucose-regulated protein 94 (GRP94), which is directly mediated by NF-κB activation to interact with HCV E2, plays an important role in TGF-protein induction, suggesting that GRP94 is a potential target for the development of drugs that prevent hepatic fibrosis caused by HCV infection. Moreover, TGF plays a pivotal role in the generation of Treg cells from precursor cells, such that a GRP94-inhibiting drug would also likely boost immunity against HCV infection by blocking the induction of Treg cells, which direct the immune tolerance against HCV [100, 101].

KCs with heme are metabolized and detoxified by heme oxygenase-1 (HMOX1) to carbon monoxide (CO), biliverdin, and free iron (which induces ferritin). The HMOX1 and metabolites of heme besides possessing anti-inflammatory and antioxidant properties have been noted to have antiviral effects in hepatitis C-infected cell lines. Additionally, these substances have been shown to enhance the response to IFN-α by restoring interferon-stimulated genes (ISGs) [102].

Only few studies on HEV-infected animals and humans have been published. But through immunohistochemistry, HEV antigens were detected mainly in KCs and liver sinusoidal endothelial cells, partially associated with hepatic lesions and infiltrates of CD3-positive cells. Since KCs and liver sinusoidal endothelial cells have antigen-presenting functions, they may also play a role in the host defense mechanisms and immunopathogenesis [103, 104].

In contrast to HBV and HCV, infection of HAV is self-limiting and does not induce chronic infectious disease. HAV reaches hepatocytes via KCs that bind complexes of HAV- and HAV-specific IgA antibodies via the Fcα receptor [105], and subsequently transfer the virus to hepatocytes. Different from HBV and HCV, HAV requires the disruption of host cell membranes to release its progeny. These dying hepatocytes may provide DAMP, which can be recognized by KCs and other intrahepatic immune cells, leading to the activation of these cells that can overcome viral immune escape and liver-intrinsic tolerogenic mechanisms [106].

2.3. Liver infection by parasites

Infection by the Echinococcus larval stages (larval echinococcoses) can affect humans [107], which are thus accidental to be intermediate hosts. Intermediate host infection occurs after the ingestion of eggs (passed out with the definitive host feces), which hatch releasing oncospheres that penetrate the intestinal wall, and then are carried by blood or lymph to organs. Lectins are central players in innate immune to pathogens. A screen among lectins known to be expressed in mammalian macrophages identified only the mouse Kupffer cells receptor (KCR; CLEC4F) as a lectin able to bind the *Echinococcus granulosus* LL [108]. KCs in particular are known to be tolerogenic, as opposed to conventional priming in the lymph nodes draining the organ [52]. Thus, the new data are consistent with the hypothesis that the LL carbohydrates are evolutionarily optimized for ensuring the clearance of shed LL particles by KCs. This hypothesis includes the possibility that KCR engagement favors the KCs release of anti-inflammatory mediators to participate in the infectious process to alleviate the liver injury [109–111].

Infection by the protozoan parasite *Entamoeba histolytica* causes hepatocyte damage in focal areas leading to amebic liver abscess (ALA). Selective depletion of KCs using liposome-entrapped clodronate or the inhibition of monocytes infiltration using CCR22/2 mice revealed that KCs and inflammatory Ly-6Chi monocytes, through producing TNF-α, are the main effector cells responsible for liver destruction during ALA [112].

KCs also represent the port of liver entry for Plasmodium and Leishmania, which parasitize KCs and then infect other liver cells [113]. Parasites enter into the skin after a mosquito bite, and the rapid migration of sporozoites allows them to escape clearance by local tissue phagocytic cells and to enter lymphatics and blood vessels. Via the blood, sporozoites rapidly reach the liver and, after gliding on HSPG in liver sinusoids, they use circumsporozoite protein (CSP) and thrombospondin-related anonymous protein (TRAP) to bind to KCs.

KCs are the potent target of *Leishmania donovani* amastigotes; early studies identified this on the basis of KCs characteristic morphology and anatomical position within the sinusoids [114, 115]. In these processes, hepatocytes infection is through KCs [116], indicating that these parasites use KCs to overcome the sinusoidal barrier and, ultimately, to infect hepatocytes. TREM2 expression by KCs appears to be an important determinant in resistance to liver-stage infection against Plasmodium parasites [117]. Once invading a hepatocyte, the parasites develop into merozoites, which will be released from the liver to infect erythrocytes [118]. Taken together, these data show that sporozoites not only use their migratory capacity to escape elimination by phagocytic and immune cells but also interact with and use KCs to increase their efficiency at infecting hepatocytes.

3. Kupffer cells in fatty liver disease

KCs have been implicated in various liver diseases with different etiologies that are associated with metabolic complications, such as over-nutrition, and may lead to fatty liver disease. Nonalcoholic fatty liver diseases (NAFLDs) are a series of disorders that include nonalcoholic fatty liver (NAFL), steatosis with inflammation, and nonalcoholic steatohepatitis. NAFLD could cause insulin resistance and is known to increase morbidity and mortality, particularly due to an increased cardiovascular risk [119–121]. KCs, liver-resident macrophages, display a critical mediator in the development of NAFLD. PAMPs and DAMPs are well known to be able to activate various Toll-like receptors (TLR) such as TLR2, 4, and 9 present on KCs, by recruiting MyD88 and engaging MAP kinases and activating NF-κB signaling, and could be responsible for the inflammatory reaction at different disease stages. Obese and steatotic patients corroborate the observation highlighting an increased CD68 mRNA of KCs with obesity, and upregulation of many other genes such as chemoattractant protein-1 (MCP-1), which is also named chemokine ligand 2 (CCL2). So CCR2-deficient animals show decreased steatosis. Soluble CD163 would also correlate with nonalcoholic fatty liver disease activity and fibrosis. Deletion of ED2-positive KCs by GdCl3 or clodronate attenuates pro-inflammatory and profibrogenic cytokines release, thereby protecting fatty livers from progression to NAFLD [122–125].

More recently, it was shown that over-expression of CD14, a coreceptor of TLR4, in KCs of mice with high-fat diet (HFD)-induced steatosis increased the hypersensitivity to low-dose LPS [126]. TLR4 in KCs mediates the progression of simple steatosis to NAFLD, by inducing ROS-dependent activation of X-box–binding protein-1 [127]. When KCs are activated by LPS through TLR4, they display an M1 TNF-expressing pro-inflammatory phenotype and increase triglyceride accumulation, decrease fatty acid oxidation and insulin responsiveness of hepatocytes. KC-derived TNF production seems to be central in NAFLD development, when silencing liver TNF or using TNFR1/2-deficient mice attenuating liver steatosis compared with wild-type mice [128, 129].

NOD-like receptors of KCs (NLRs) are intracellular PRRs that are part of the inflammasomes briefly mentioned above. Inflammasomes are multiprotein complexes that through NLRs sense intracellular danger signals and initiate an activation cascade of events that culminate with autoactivation of caspase 1 and cleavage of promoting IL-1κ and IL-18 production. By controlling the release of these important inflammatory cytokines, inflammasomes play an important role in the inflammatory process underlying NAFLD [130].

Interestingly, it was recently shown that IL-10 released by activated KCs stimulated apoptotic death of pro-inflammatory cells [131]. This mechanism mediated resistance to hepatocyte steatosis and subsequently death. Fatty liver disease mechanism caused by excessive alcohol consumption is similar as NAFLD. In the same way, the depletion of KCs in mice also attenuates alcohol-induced diseases. Then it demonstrated a central role of KCs in fatty liver diseases [132].

4. Kupffer cells in liver fibrosis

Fibrogenesis development has many pathological factors, such as inflammation derived from Kupffer cells, angiogenesis, and hepatic stellate cell (HSC) activation, and interacts with each other, leading to collagen deposition. Cirrhosis is the most advanced stage of fibrosis, with septa and nodule formation being the most notable features [133]. KCs or resident hepatic macrophages carry out an important role in modulating inflammation in liver fibrosis development. KCs produce reactive oxygen species, a variety of pro-inflammatory cytokines, such as TNF-α, IL-1β, and macrophage inflammatory protein (MIP)-1, which could provoke HSC activation to produce pro-fibrotic cytokines TGF-β and platelet-derived growth factor (PDGF) and subsequently contribute to hepatic injury [134, 135].

The accumulation of circulating Ly6Chi monocytes within the liver is greatly dependent on CCR2/CCL2 and CCL1/CCR8 axis, in the pathogenesis process, KCs also express multiple chemokines and matrix metalloproteinases (MMP-9, -12, and -13) that recruit immune cells and promote extracellular matrix degradation, thus favoring the resolution of fibrosis [136]. Then, senescent hepatocytes and NF-κB-inducing kinase (NIK) activation in hepatocytes lead to the release of numerous chemokines. These chemokines can influence the migration or activation state of macrophages that in turn induce hepatocyte apoptosis. Accordingly, the NIK in vivo triggers massive liver inflammation and hepatocyte apoptosis leading to liver fibrosis. The fact that on the basis of above experiments KCs depletion using clodronate reversed NIK-induced damage [137, 138].

Some studies indicate that activating CX3CR1 on KCs increases their IL-10 expression and reduces their TNF and TGF-β [139], IL-10 is a potent anti-inflammatory mediator that has been shown to inhibit the production of TNF-α and IL-1 and to suppress the activation of NF-κB . IL-10 reduces macrophage production of nitric oxide (NO) and reactive oxygen intermediates, and also reduces the expression of adhesion molecules and chemokines [140, 141]. Thus, fractalkine (the ligand of CX3CR1) represents a negative feedback on the extension of liver inflammation through affecting KCs.

An antifibrotic effect of liver macrophages was also demonstrated when macrophage infiltration was blocked during the induction of fibrogenesis in rats. Delta-like ligand 4 (Dll4) is a kind of antifibrotic factor. It was expressed in patients' KCs and liver sinusoidal endothelial cells.

In vitro, rDll4 significantly decreased lipopolysaccharide-dependent chemokine expression in both KCs and HSCs. Then the inflammatory cell infiltration and their chemokine ligand 2 (CCL2) expression were significantly reduced in rDll4-receiving bile duct ligation mice. Dll4 expression was inversely associated with CCL2 abundance. Mechanistically, Dll4 regulated CCL2 expression via NF-κB. Taken together, Dll4 modulates liver inflammatory response by downregulating chemokine expression and then participates in the role of antifibrosis of liver [142, 143]. With regard to recovery from fibrosis, KCs and macrophages secrete proteinases that promote the degradation of scarring extracellular matrix proteins.

5. Kupffer cells in liver ischemia-reperfusion injury

Liver ischemia reperfusion (I/R) injury refers to the paradoxic aggravation of ischemic liver resulting from the return of blood flow and oxygen delivery, which is encountered frequently in a variety of clinical situations, including liver transplantation, trauma, hepatic resection, or hypovolemic shock. If hepatic I/R injury progresses out of control, it can lead to liver failure, systemic inflammatory response syndrome, and multiple organ failure, and lastly leading to death [144, 145]. Oxidative stress is the major contributor for I/R-induced injury, so the therapeutic strategies to antioxidants have gained interest. In I/R injury, KC activation is presumed to occur first, resulting in generation of reactive oxygen species (ROS) and preinflammatory cytokines such as TNF-α, IL-1β, nitric oxide, and chemokines, which contribute to hepatocyte death, endothelial damage and recruitment, and activation of leukocytes [146].

KCs secrete CCL2 to promote CCR2-expressing neutrophil recruitment from the bone marrow and subsequent infiltration into the liver during I/R [147], and secrete matrix metalloproteinases (MMPs) to increase graft dysfunction [148]. In this process, platelets could be adherent to the KCs, which reflect the activation of KCs and lead to leukocyte accumulation affecting sinusoidal perfusion, causing liver failure [149].

Large amounts of endotoxin contact KCs through the portal circulation following IR after liver transplantation. The LPS first binds to CD14, triggering KCs activation, then integrates with TLR4, and further increases the expression of CD14, the activation signals are transduced into cytoplasm, resulting in NF-κB nuclear translocation and cytokines such as TNF-α and IL-6 release, harming the liver graft. TLR4 knockout mice are protected from endothelial overactivation in the absence of KCs after IR injury [150]. At the same time, endoplasmic reticulum (ER) stress of KCs in evoking liver inflammation following reperfusion contributed to the conversion of natural Tregs to Th17 cells due to IL-6 release, resulting in liver injury [151]. Whereas the inhibition of high-mobility group box 1 production by KCs after I/R in rats could prevent liver injury [152], suppression of TNF-α–mediated apoptotic signaling by glutathione (GSH) pretreatment can attenuate hepatic I/R injury in young and aged rats [153].

In IR injury, activated KCs could produce pro-inflammation cytokine IL-18, blocking of IL-18 by IL-18-binding protein may inhibit KCs activation, resulting in a reduction of KC-derived harmful stimuli, then ameliorates I/R injury [154]. KCs also could protect liver grafts against liver-transplant–induced I/R injury. The protection appears to be mediated by the release

http://dx.doi.org/10.5772/67673

of anti-inflammatory IL-10 and the production of antioxidant heme oxygenase by KCs [41, 155]. The IL-10 secreted by KCs controls pro-inflammatory mediators released from LSEC in response to LPS challenge, KCs depletion has also been shown to impair hepatic IL-10 production after partial hepatectomy. Pretreatment with IL-10 protects steatotic livers undergoing I/R, and that active KCs retain a hepatoprotective role in the steatotic environment [156, 157].

Heme oxygenase-1 (HO-1) is a rate-limiting enzyme of heme degradation, exerts antioxidative, antiapoptotic, anti-inflammatory, and vasoactive effects through its byproducts or itself. HO-1 and its byproducts (CO, biliverdin, and iron ion) induction could protect the graft from IR injury after liver transplantation in several experimental studies [158]. Our study also has the same results. Our results of immunofluorescence also demonstrated that preconditioning with Nodosin perfusion induced HO-1 expression mainly in KCs at 24 h after transplantation [159] (**Figure 3**). HO-1 upregulation in KCs plays a protective role in modulating immune responses of I/R-injured tissues, or reducing apoptosis induced directly by TNF-α [160]. Preincubation of KCs with CO upregulated heat-shock protein 70 (HSP70) and inhibited ROS generation. CO-pretreated liver grafts showed less upregulation of TNF-α and inducible nitric oxide synthase messenger RNA (mRNA), reduced expression of pro-apoptotic B cell lymphoma 2-associated X protein mRNA, cleaved caspase-3, and poly(adenosine diphosphate ribose) polymerase. So, pretreatment of donors with CO ameliorates LT-associated I/R injury with increased hepatic HSP70 expression, particularly in the KCs population [161].

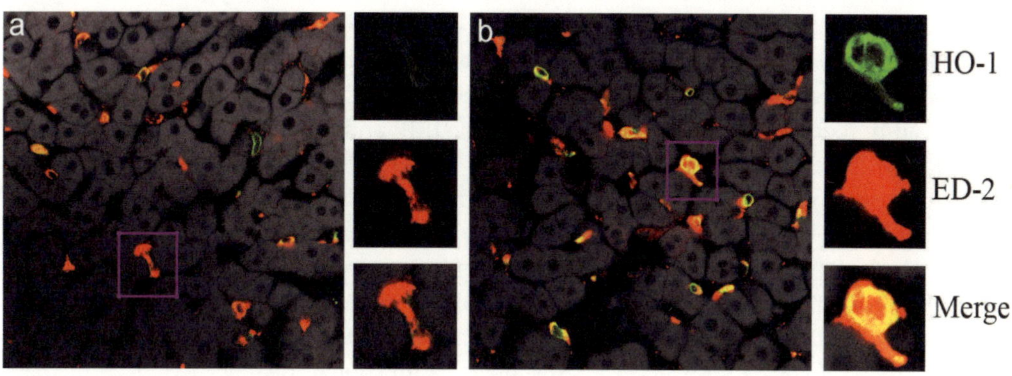

Figure 3. Immunofluorescence double staining for cellular localization of heme oxygenase 1 (HO-1) expression in the rat liver after nodosin perfusion. Liver sections are stained for HO-1 (green) and the Kupffer cell marker ED2 (red). Colocalization of these two colors can be recognized by the yellow color. (a) Control group; (b) *Nodosin* group; (x40) [165].

6. Kupffer cells in liver transplantation immunology

Liver transplantation is an effective treatment for advanced liver diseases, but immune rejection is a major obstacle after transplantation. KCs not only can engulf and kill pathogenic microorganisms, rid of endotoxin, but also have effects of antigen presentation, secretion of cytokines, and immune regulation. They can express high levels of MHC and costimulatory molecules and are capable of activating naive T cells [17]. At the same time, they could be activated by antigen to produce T1 cytokines IL-2, IL-1, IL-6, TNF-α, and IFN-γ. They interact with the recipient T cells that migrate into the graft and play an important role in immune response [162]. Furthermore, the replacement of KCs by recipient bone marrow-derived cells (BMDCs) was observed in the liver graft, and functional inhibition of KCs by GdCl3 abrogated prolonged survival. Analysis of mRNA expression levels in liver grafts showed a shift of the Th1/Th2 balance toward reducing rejection in the BMC groups. So replacement of KCs by recipient BMDCs may play an important role in this mechanism of inhibiting rejection [163].

After liver transplantation, the reduction of B7 expression in donor KCs could suppress the activation of recipient T lymphocytes and secretion of IL-2 via the CD28/B7 costimulatory pathway and may induce immune tolerance [164]. The cytokines TNF-α expression in KCs is a marker of activated KCs after transplantation and it may be a good target for reversing acute rejection post transplantation [165]. GdCl3 depletion of KCs also plays a protective role in liver transplantation through suppressing bile duct cell apoptosis, including decreasing expression of ALT, ALP, TBIL, and TNF-α, and suppressing Fas-FasL-Caspase signal transduction [166].

KCs not only play a role in immune response directly but also activate the immature DCs or recruit immature DCs to liver to mature DCs to take part in immune response, by producing pro-inflammation cytokines and chemokines .Then, mDCs could express costimulatory molecules highly and present antigen to T cells [167, 168].

Recently, it has found that KCs can induce T lymphocyte apoptosis and play an important role in the regulation of liver transplantation tolerance. They also could produce high levels of Th2 cytokines IL-10 and TGF-β and low levels of IL-12 to protect the graft [169]. Although KCs can promote immature DCs to mature DCs as immunogenic APCs, they are frequently accompanied by an upregulation of PD-L1 [170], release of IL-10 and TGF-β [171], prostaglandin E2 (PGE2) [172], IDO [173, 174] and/or arginase [175], which inhibit DC-mediated T cell activation within the sinusoids, and the presentation of high-affinity peptide by KCs results in the deletion of $CD8^+$ T cell tolerance. Furthermore, they promote the suppressive capacity of Tregs ($CD4^+CD25^+FoxP3^+$ T cells) toward hepatic antigens to induce tolerance [176]. KCs could also recruit TH17 cells and also $\gamma\delta$ T cells are facilitated by CCR6 and possibly also CCR4 via CCL17, CCL22, and CCL20. A broad variety of chemokine receptors have been linked to Treg cell migration (e.g., CCR1, CCR4, CCR5, and CCR6) showing a functional tolerance [28]. KCs mediate $CD8^+$ T cells apoptosis by expressing Fas ligand (FasL), which can ligate Fas on $CD8^+$ T cells [177]. V-set and Ig domain-containing 4 (VSIG4, CRIg, or Z39Ig), a newly identified B7-related cosignaling molecule, exclusive expression on liver KCs is a complement receptor for C3b and iC3b and a coinhibitory ligand that negatively regulates T-cell immunity, $VSIG4^+$ KCs play a critical role in the induction and maintenance of liver T- and NKT-cell tolerance [178]. So, KCs have a dual effect after liver transplantation immunology

7. Kupffer cells in liver cancer and metastases

Persistent hepatic inflammation resulting from hepatitis B or C virus infections (HBV or HCV, respectively), NAFLD, or alcohol abuse is a hallmark feature of chronic liver diseases and appears to be an essential prerequisite of hepatocarcinogenesis. The results of this activation involve the production of multiple inflammatory cytokines, ROS, growth control mediators, various chemokines, which orchestrate the interaction between parenchymal and nonparenchymal liver cells, especially KCs to be activated in the process of hepatic carcinogenesis. They are also involved in the enhancement of clonal expansion of preneoplastic cells, then leading to neoplasia [179]. In diethylnitrosamine-induced HCC in mice, pro-inflammatory activation of KCs during the early stages of chemical-induced carcinogenesis is important in tumor development. Then, the antitumor effects of KCs are widely studied, such as to release TNF-α and iNO to recruit cytotoxic T cells and NK cells, to induce apoptosis of cancer cells and phagocytose cancer cells [180]. And some studies demonstrated that the expression of TREM-1 by mouse KCs plays a crucial role in their activation upon the recognition of necrotic hepatocytes and tumor cells [181]. Activated KCs suppress tumor cells through the ADCC pathway via FcγRIII (CD16) and directly or indirectly by cytokines. The existence of CD16a in KCs and that the activation of KCs, which mainly resulted in CD16a expression, then via NK cells, mediated ADCC reactions to induce NK cell cytotoxicity to tumor cells.

The activated KCs kill target cells directly by swallowing and releasing lysosomal enzyme, NO, and peroxidase; they also cooperate to resist tumor cells by secreting cytokines including TNF-α, IL-1, IL-6, and granulocyte-macrophage colony-stimulating factor (GM-CSF) [182, 183]. IL-6 is highly produced by KCs, it has been related with tumor progression and angiogenesis in several tumors, and it is overproduced in HCC. So decreasing the IL-6 production by KCs inhibits hepatocellular carcinoma growths [184]. KCs derived from male but not female SART1+/− mice produced increased levels of the hypoxia inducible factor (HIF-1)-dependent chemokine (RANTES) and cytokine promoting oxidative damage and inflammation, driving progression to hepatocellular carcinoma. Reventing inappropriate HIF-1 activation in male mice, as a novel therapeutic target for hepatocellular carcinoma [185, 186].

KCs play an essential function in the host tumoral surveillance system. Their strategic position in liver allows them to discriminate and remove neoplastic cells that develop in liver. Besides primary liver cancer, liver metastases are frequently observed, especially in gastrointestinal malignancies. The metastatic cells migrate via the bloodstream into the portal circulation, and they are entrapped in the liver sinusoids [187]. KCs play an important role in tumor growth, angiogenesis, and metastasis through the production of a number of growth factors (PDGF-β, vascular endothelial growth factor (VEGF), TGF-β, and EGFR ligands), cytokines (IL-6, TNFα, and IL-10), chemokines (CCL17, CCL22, CCL24, CXCL12, and IL-8), as well as other soluble factors (MMPs, osteopontin, and cyclooxyganse-2). In the liver, CEA binds with heterogeneous nuclear RNA-binding protein M (hnRNP M) receptor on KCs and causes activation and production of pro- and anti-inflammatory cytokines including IL-1, IL-10, IL-6, and TNF-α. These cytokines affect the upregulation of adhesion molecules on the hepatic sinusoidal endothelium and protect the tumor cells against cytotoxicity by nitric oxide (NO) and other reactive oxygen radicals. This activation is the key to the role of CEA in liver metastasis. A large number of clinical studies have shown correlations between serum CEA levels and advanced colorectal cancer, in particular, in the presence of liver metastasis [188].

KCs were found to have promoted tumor invasion and exacerbated the metastasis and they are responsible for the accumulation of liposomes. In the metastatic hepatic cancer, KCs taking up liposomes were significantly increased, and PEGylated can reverse this result through a reduction in tumor-supportive KCs [189]. Primary pancreatic tumor cells release exosomes that contain migration inhibitory factor (MIF) into the blood circulation. These PDAC-derived exosomes are selectively taken up by liver KCs, leading to the MIF-dependent production of fibrotic cytokines by KCs. These fibrotic cytokines, particularly TGF-β, activate liver HSCs to produce fibronectin. Deposition of fibronectin in the liver leads to the formation of a fibrotic microenvironment that promotes the recruitment of bone marrow-derived cells. These sequential events establish a premetastatic niche, which permits the survival and proliferation of disseminated PDAC cells and the formation of metastases in the liver [190]. Some studies demonstrated that KCs could help metastatic cancer cells extravasate from vessel via CXCL12/CXCR4 pathway.

KCs in liver can interact with myeloid-derived suppressor cells (MDSCs) and cause their upregulation of PD-L1, a negative T cell costimulatory molecule, and ultimately lead to tumor immunosuppression in accordance with further tumor progression and metastasis. They can suppress $CD8^+$ T cells function via B7-H1/programmed death-1 interactions, which diminishes antitumor effect of $CD8^+$ T cells. The metastatic tumor cells entering the liver from portal vein triggered KCs and mediated also upregulation of vascular endothelial cell adhesion receptors, such as E-selectin to help metastatic tumor cells arrest and extravasate [191–193]. KCs themselves are controversial, in metastatic colon tumors, the cytokines produced by KCs (IL-12 and IFN-α) are indeed important for the activation of NK cells and NKT cells and for preventing tumor liver metastases, depletion of KCs by gadolinium chloride or clodronate liposomes increased the number of liver metastasis in some reports [194]. Other studies have demonstrated that KCs induce Fas expression in colon cancer cells and malignant glioma cells leading to Fas-mediated apoptosis and death in the presence of tumor-infiltrating lymphocytes or TNF-α [195].

8. Conclusion

Kupffer cells have various functions in liver injury and repair. KCs, as liver-resident macrophages, localize within the lumen of the liver sinusoids and are adherent to the endothelial cells that compose the blood vessel walls. They are the first immune cells in the liver that come in contact with the gut bacteria, gut bacterial endotoxins, and microbial debris derived from the gastrointestinal tract that have been transported to the liver via the portal vein. They also interact with other hepatic cells to play an essential role in the host defense. They are responsible for the development of liver diseases including infectious disease, fatty liver disease, liver fibrosis and cirrhosis, ischemia and reperfusion injury, liver transplantation immunology as well as liver cancer. But KCs express various phenotypes to have various functions. Because of the highly overlapping characteristics of these cells, their functions are controversial. The complex roles of KCs in both protective and harmful responses make the liver diseases treatment interesting but difficult. So, further efforts should therefore focus on regulatory mechanisms in specific subpopulations of KCs differentiation and function.

http://dx.doi.org/10.5772/67673

Acknowledgements

The authors thank the National Natural Science Foundation of China (grant nos. 81270555 and 81470897) and the Program for New Century Excellent Talents in University (grant no. NECT-13-0422) for their support.

Author details

Yuan-yuan Ma[1], Mu-qing Yang[2], Zhi-gang He[2], Qing Wei[1] and Ji-yu Li[2]*

*Address all correspondence to: leejiyu@sina.com

1 Department of Pathology, Shanghai Tenth People's Hospital, Tongji University, Shanghai, PR China

2 Department of General Surgery, Shanghai Tenth People's Hospital, Tongji University, Shanghai, PR China

References

[1] Duarte N, Coelho IC, Patarrão RS, et al. How inflammation impinges on NAFLD: a role for Kupffer cells. BioMed Res Int. 2015:984578. doi:10.1155/2015/984578.

[2] Gomez P, Klapproth K, Schulz CE, et al. Tissue-resident macrophages originate from yolk-sac-derived erythro-myeloid progenitors. Nature. 2015;518(7540):547–551. doi:10.1038/nature13989.

[3] Ramachandran P, Pellicoro A, Vernon MA, et al. Differential Ly-6C expression identifies the recruited macrophage phenotype, which orchestrates the regression of murine liver fibrosis. Proc Natl Acad Sci USA. 2012;109:E3186–E3195. doi:10.1073/pnas.1119964109.

[4] Schulz C, Gomez PE, Chorro L, et al. A lineage of myeloid cells independent of Myb and hematopoietic stem cells. Science. 2012;336(6077):86–90. doi:10.1126/science.1219179.

[5] Tacke F, Zimmermann HW, et al. Macrophage heterogeneity in liver injury and fibrosis. J Hepatol. 2014;60(5):1090–1096. doi:10.1016/j.jhep.2013.12.025.

[6] Zimmermann HW, Trautwein C, Tacke F, et al. Functional role of monocytes and macrophages for the inflammatory response in acute liver injury. Front Physiol. 2012;3:56. doi:10.3389/fphys.2012.00056.

[7] Bain CC, Bravo-Blas A, Scott CL, et al. Constant replenishment from circulating monocytes maintains the macrophage pool in the intestine of adult mice. Nat Immunol. 2014;15(10):929–937. doi:10.1038/ni.2967.

[8] Yona S, Kim KW, Wolf Y, et al. Fate mapping reveals origins and dynamics of monocytes and tissue macrophages under homeostasis. Immunity. 2013;38(1):79–91. doi:10.1016/j.immuni.2012.12.001.

[9] Guilliams M, De Kleer I, Henri S, et al. Alveolar macrophages develop from fetal monocytes that differentiate into long-lived cells in the first week of life via GM-CSF. J Exp Med. 2013;210(10):1977–1992. doi:10.1084/jem.20131199.

[10] Hoeffel G, Wang Y, Greter M, et al. Adult Langerhans cells derive predominantly from embryonic fetal liver monocytes with a minor contribution of yolk sac-derived macrophages. J Exp Med. 2012;209(6):1167–1181. doi:10.1084/jem.20120340.

[11] Hoeffel G, Chen J, Lavin Y, et al. C-myb(þ) erythro-myeloid progenitor-derived fetal monocytes give rise to adult tissue-resident macrophages. Immunity. 2015;42(4):665–678. doi:10.1016/j.immuni.2015.03.011.

[12] Charlotte LS, Fang Z, Patrick De B, et al. Bone marrow-derived monocytes give rise to self-renewing and fully differentiated Kupffer cells. Nat Commun. 2016;7:10321. doi:10.1038/ncomms10321.

[13] Naito M, Hasegawa G, Ebe Y, et al. Differentiation and function of Kupffer cells. Med Electron Microsc. 2014;37(1):16–28. doi:10.1007/s00795-003-0228-x.

[14] Xing XK, Wu HY, Feng HG, et al. Immune function of nonparenchymal liver cells. Genet Mol Res 2016;15(1):gmr.15018524. doi:10.4238/gmr.15018524.

[15] Heymann F, Tacke F, et al. Immunology in the liver -from homeostasis to disease Nat Rev Gastroenterol Hepatol. 2016;13(2):88–110. doi:10.1038/nrgastro.2015.200.

[16] Hashimoto D, Chow A, Noizat C, et al. Tissue- resident macrophages self-maintain locally throughout adult life with minimal contribution from circulating monocytes. Immunity. 2013;38(4):792–804. doi:10.1016/j.immuni.2013.04.004.

[17] Kinoshita M, Uchida T, Sato A, et al. Characterization of two F4/80-positive Kupffer cell subsets by their function and phenotype in mice. J Hepatol. 2010;53(5):903–910. doi:10.1016/j.jhep.2010.04.037.

[18] Bouwens L, Baekeland M, De Zanger R, et al. Quantitation, tissue distribution and proliferation kinetics of Kupffer cells in normal rat liver. Hepatology. 1986;6(4):718–722. doi:10.1002/hep.1840060430.

[19] Laskin DL, Weinberger B, Laskin JD, et al. Functional heterogeneity in liver and lung macrophages. J Leukoc Biol. 2001;70(2):163–170.

[20] Horst AK, Neumann K, Diehl L, et al. Modulation of liver tolerance by conventional and nonconventional antigen-presenting cells and regulatory immune cells. Cell Mol. Immunol. 2016;13(3):277–292. doi:10.1038/cmi.2015.112.

[21] Nascimento M, Huang SC, Smith A, et al. Ly6Chi monocyte recruitment is responsible for Th2 associated host-protective macrophage accumulation in liver inflammation due to schistosomiasis. PLoS Pathog. 2014;10:e1004282. doi:10.1371/journal.ppat.1004282.

[22] Zigmond E, Samia-Grinberg S, Pasmanik-Chor M, et al. Infiltrating monocyte-derived macrophages and resident Kupffer cells display different ontogeny and functions in acute liver injury. J Immunol. 2014;193(1):344–353. doi:10.4049/jimmunol.1400574.

[23] Davies LC, Jenkins SJ, Allen JE, et al. Tissue-resident macrophages. Nat Immunol. 2013;14:986–995. doi:10.1038/ni.2705.

[24] Breous E, Somanathan S, Vandenberghe LH, et al. Hepatic regulatory T cells and Kupffer cells are crucial mediators of systemic T cell tolerance to antigens targeting murine liver. Hepatology. 2009;50(2):612–621. doi:10.1002/hep.23043.

[25] Lavin Y, Winter D, Blecher-Gonen R, et al. Tissue-resident macrophage enhancer landscapes are shaped by the local microenvironment. Cell. 2014;159(6):1312–1326. doi:10.1016/j.cell.2014.11.018.

[26] Gautier EL, Shay T, Miller J, et al. Gene-expression profiles and transcriptional regulatory pathways that underlie the identity and diversity of mouse tissue macrophages. Nat Immunol. 2012;13(1):1118–1128. doi:10.1038/ni.2419.

[27] Yang C-Y, Chen J-B, Tsai T-F, et al. CLEC4F is an inducible C-type lectin in F4/80-positive cells and is involved in alpha-galactosylceramide presentation in liver. PLoS One. 2013;8:e65070. doi:10.1371/journal.pone.0065070.

[28] Heymann F, Peusquens J, Ludwig-Portugall I, et al. Liver inflammation abrogates immunological tolerance induced by Kupffer cells. Hepatology. 2015;62(1):279–291. doi:10.1002/hep.27793.

[29] Deshane J, Wright M, Agarwal A, et al. Heme oxygenase-1 expression in disease states. Acta Biochim Pol. 2005;52(2):273–284.

[30] Kikumi S, Ozaki S, Kimura N, et al. Use of carbon monoxide in minimizing ischemia/reperfusion injury in transplantation. Transplant Rev. 2012;26(2):125–139. doi:10.1016/j.trre.2011.01.004.

[31] Ellett JD, Atkinson C, Evans ZP, et al. Toll-like receptor 4 knockout mice are protected from endothelial overactivation in the absence of Kupffer cells after total hepatic ischemia/reperfusion. Liver Transpl. 2011;17(9):1089–1098. doi:10.1002/lt.22333.

[32] Wu J, Meng Z, Jiang M, et al. Hepatitis B virus suppresses toll-like receptor mediated innate immune responses in murine parenchymal and non-parenchymal liver cells. Hepatology. 2009;49(4):1132–1140. doi:10.1002/hep.22751.

[33] Visvanathan K, Skinner NA, Thompson AJ, et al. Regulation of toll-like receptor-2 expression in chronic hepatitis B by the precore protein. Hepatology. 2007;45(1):102–110. doi:10.1002/hep.21482.

[34] Takii Y, Nakamura M, Ito M, et al. Enhanced expression of type I interferon and toll-like receptor-3 in primary biliary cirrhosis. Lab. Invest. 2005;85(7):908–920. doi:10.1038/labinvest.3700285.

[35] Imaizumi T, Sashinami H, Mori F, et al. Listeria monocyto- genes induces the expression of retinoic acid-inducible gene-I. Microbiol Immunol. 2006;50(10):811–815. doi:10.1111/j.1348-0421.2006.tb03857.

[36] Body-Malapel M, Dharancy S, Berrebi D, et al. NOD2: a potential target for regulating liver injury. Lab Invest. 2008;88(3):318–327. doi:10.1038/labinvest.3700716.

[37] Su GL. Lipopolysaccharides in liver injury: molecular mechanisms of Kupffer cell activation. Am J Physiol. 2002;283(2):G256–G265. doi:10.1152/ajpgi.00550.2001.

[38] Ferrero E, Jiao D, Tsuberi BZ, et al. Transgenic mice expressing human CD14 are hypersensitive to lipopolysaccharide. Proc Natl Acad Sci USA. 1993;90(6):2380–2384.

[39] Tu Z, Bozorgzadeh A, Pierce RH, et al. TLR-dependent cross talk between human Kupffer cells and NK cells. J Exp Med. 2008;205(1):233–244. doi:10.1084/jem.20072195.

[40] Boltjes A, Movita D, Boonstra A, et al. The role of Kupffer cells in hepatitis B and hepatitis C virus infection. J Hepatol. 2014;61(3):660–671. doi:10.1016/j.jhep.2014.04.026.

[41] Bamboat ZM, Ocuin LM, Balachandran VP, et al. Conventional DCs reduce liver ischemia/reperfusion injury in mice via IL-10 secretion. J Clin Invest. 2010;120(2):559–569. doi:10.1172/JCI40008.

[42] Szabo G, Csak T. Inflammasomes in liver diseases. J Hepatol. 2012;57(3):642–654. doi:10.1016/j.jhep.2012.03.035.

[43] Elsegood CL, Chan CW, Degli-Esposti MA, et al. Kupffer cell-monocyte communication is essential for initiating murine liver progenitor cell-mediated liver regeneration. Hepatology. 2015;62(4):1272–1284. doi:10.1002/hep.27977.

[44] Seki E, De MS, Osterreicher CH, et al. TLR4 enhances TGF-beta signaling and hepatic fibrosis. Nat Med. 2007;13(1):1324–1332. doi:10.1038/nm1663.

[45] Hemmi H, Kaisho T, Takeuchi O, et al. Small anti-viral compounds activate immune cells via the TLR7 MyD88-dependent signaling pathway. Nat Immunol. 2002;3(2):196–200. doi:10.1038/ni758.

[46] Mosser DM, Edwards JP. Exploring the full spectrum of macrophage activation. Nat Rev Immunol. 2008;8(12):958–969. doi:10.1038/nri2448.

[47] Hutchinson JA, Riquelme P, Sawitzki B, et al. Cutting edge: immunological consequences and trafficking of human regulatory macrophages administered to renal transplant recipients. J Immunol. 2011;187(5):2072–2078. doi:10.4049/jimmunol.1100762.

[48] Vollmar B, Menger MD. The hepatic microcirculation: mechanistic contributions and therapeutic targets in liver injury and repair. Physiol Rev. 2009;89(4):1269–1339. doi:10.1152/physrev.00027.2008.

[49] Rutella S, Bonanno G, Procoli A, et al. Hepatocyte growth factor favors monocyte differentiation into regulatory interleukin (IL)-10++IL-12low/neg accessory cells with dendritic-cell features. Blood. 2006;108(1):218–227. doi:10.1182/blood-2005-08-3141.

[50] Li G, Kim YJ, Broxmeyer HE. Macrophage colony-stimulating factor drives cord blood monocyte differentiation into IL-10highIL-12absent dendritic cells with tolerogenic potential. J Immunol. 2005;174(8):4706–4717. doi:10.4049/ jimmunol.174.8.4706.

[51] Crispe IN. The liver as a lymphoid organ. Annu Rev Immunol. 2009;27:147–163. doi:10.1146/annurev.immunol.021908.132629.

[52] Thomson AW, Knolle PA. Antigen-presenting cell function in the tolerogenic liver environment. Nat Rev Immunol. 2010;10(11):753–766. doi:10.1038/nri2858.

[53] Kedarisetty CK, Anand L, Bhardwaj A, et al. Combination of granulocyte colony-stimulating factor and erythropoietin improves outcomes of patients with decompensated cirrhosis. Gastroenterology. 2015;148(7):1362–1370.e7. doi:10.1053/j.gastro.2015.02.054.

[54] Geissmann F, Cameron TO, Sidobre S, et al. Intravascular immune surveillance by CXCR6+ NKT cells patrolling liver sinusoids. PLoS Biol. 2005;3(4):e113. doi:10.1371/journal.pbio.0030113.

[55] Wehr A, Baeck C, Heymann F, et al. Chemokine receptor CXCR6-dependent hepatic NK T cell accumulation promotes inflammation and liver fibrosis. J Immunol. 2013; 190(10):5226–5236. doi:10.4049/jimmunol.1202909.

[56] Trobonjaca Z, Leithäuser F, Möller P, et al. Activating immunity in the liver. I. Liver dendritic cells (but not hepatocytes) are potent activators of IFN-γ release by liver NKT cells. J Immunol. 2001;167(3):1413–1422. doi:10.4049/ jimmunol.167.3.1413.

[57] Schmieg J, Yang G, Franck R, et al. Glycolipid presentation to natural killerT cells differs in an organ-dependent fashion.Proc Natl Acad Sci USA. 2005;102(4):1127–1132. doi:10.1073/pnas.0408288102.

[58] Lee WY, Moriarty TJ, Wong CH, et al. An intravascular immune response to *Borrelia burgdorferi* involves Kupffer cells and iNKT cells. Nat Immunol. 2010;11(4):295–302. doi:10.1038/ni.1855.

[59] Beattie L, Phillips R, Brown N, et al. Interferon regulatory factor 7 contributes to the control of *Leishmania donovani* in the mouse liver. Infect Immun. 2011;79(3):1057–1066. doi:10.1128/IAI.00633-10.

[60] Tay SS, Wong YC, Roediger B, et al. Intrahepatic activation of naive CD4+ T cells by liver-resident phagocytic cells. J Immunol. 2014;193(5):2087–2095. doi:10.4049/jimmunol.1400037.

[61] Afford SC, Humphreys EH, Reid DT, et al. Vascular cell adhesion molecule 1 expression by biliary epithelium promotes persistence of inflammation by inhibiting effector T-cell apoptosis. Hepatology. 2014;59(5):1932–1943. doi:10.1002/hep.26965.

[62] Watanabe Y, Morita M, Ikematsu N, et al. Tumor necrosis factor a and interleukin-1β but not interferon induce vascular cell adhesion molecule-1 expression on primary cultured murine hepatocytes. Biochem Biophys Res Commun. 1995;209:335–342. doi:10.1006/bbrc.1995.1508.

[63] John B, Crispe IN. Passive and active mechanisms trap activated CD8+ T cells in the liver. J Immunol. 2004;172(9):5222–5229. doi:10.4049/ jimmunol.172.9.5222.

[64] Morita M, Watanabe Y, Akaike T. Inflammatory cytokines up- regulate intercellular adhesion molecule-1 expression on primary cultured mouse hepatocytes and T-lymphocyte adhesion. Hepatology. 1994;19(2):426–431. doi:10.1002/hep.1840190222.

[65] Muehlen KA, Schuemann J, Wittke F, et al. NK cells, but not NKT cells, are involved in *Pseudomonas aeruginosa* exotoxin A-induced hepatotoxicity in mice. J Immunol. 2004;172(5):3034–3041. doi:10.4049/ jimmunol.172.5.3034.

[66] Oosten MV, Bilt EVD, Vries HED, et al. Vascular adhesion molecule-1 and intercellular adhesion molecule-1 expression on rat liver cells after lipopolysaccharide administration in vivo. Hepatology. 1995;22(5):1538–1546. doi:10.1002/hep.1840220529.

[67] Wiiluweit A, Sass G, Sch€oneberg A, et al. Chronic inflammation and protection from acute hepatitis in transgenic mice expressing TNF in endothelial cells. J Immunol. 2001;167(7):3944–3952. doi:10.4049/ jimmunol.167.7.3944.

[68] Okada T, Kimura A, Kanki K, et al. Liver resident macrophages (Kupffer cells) share several functional antigens in common with endothelial cells. Scand J Immunol. 2016;83(2):139–150. doi:10.1111/sji.12402.

[69] Xu R, Huang H, Zhang Z, et al. The role of neutrophils in the development of liver diseases. Cell Mol Immunol. 2014;11(3):224–231. doi:10.1038/cmi.2014.2.

[70] Ramadori G, Moriconi F, Malik I, et al. Physiology and pathophysiology of liver inflammation, damage and repair. J Physiol Pharmacol 2008;59:S107–S117.

[71] Disson O, Grayo S, Huillet E, et al. Conjugated action of two species-specific invasion proteins for fetoplacental listeriosis. Nature. 2008;455(7216):1114–1118. doi:10.1038/nature07303.

[72] Serbina NV, Pamer EG. Monocyte emigration from bone marrow during bacterial infection requires signals mediated by chemokine receptor CCR2. Nat Immunol. 2006;7(3):311–317. doi:10.1038/ni1309.

[73] Shi C, Velá zquez P, Hohl TM, et al. Monocyte trafficking to hepatic sites of bacterial infection is chemokine independent and directed by focal intercellular adhesion molecule-1 expression. J Immunol. 2010;184(11):6266–6274. doi:10.4049/jimmunol.0904160.

[74] Shi C, Hohl TM, Leiner I, et al. Ly6G+ neutrophils are dispensable for defense against systemic *Listeria monocytogenes* infection. J Immunol. 2011;187(10):5293–5298. doi:10.4049/jimmunol.1101721.

[75] Jenkins SJ, Ruckerl D, Cook PC, et al. Local macrophage proliferation, rather than recruitment from the blood, is a signature of TH2 inflammation. Science. 2011;332(6035):1284–1288. doi:10.1126/science.1204351.

[76] Ebe Y, Hasegawa G, Takatsuka H, et al. The role of Kupffer cells and regulation of neutrophil migration into the liver by macrophage inflammatory protein-2 in primary listeriosis in mice. Pathol Int. 1999;49(6):519–532. doi:10.1046/j.1440-1827.1999.00910

[77] Salkowski CA, Detore G, Franks A, et al. Pulmonary and hepatic gene expression following cecal ligation and puncture: monophosphoryl lipid A prophylaxis attenuates sepsis-induced cytokine and chemokine expression and neutrophil infiltration. Infect Immun.1998;66(8):3569–3578.

[78] Pecaric-Petkovic T, Didichenko SA, Kaempfer S, et al. Human basophils and eosinophils are the direct target leukocytes of the novel IL-1 family member IL-33. Blood. 2009;113(7):1526–1534. doi:10.1182/blood-2008-05-157818.

[79] Blériot C, Dupuis T, Jouvion G, et al. Liver-resident macrophage necroptosis orchestrates type 1 microbicidal inflammation and type-2-mediated tissue repair during bacterial infection. Immunity. 2015;42(1):145–158. doi:10.1016/j.immuni.2014.12.020.

[80] Molawi K, Sieweke MH. Monocytes compensate Kupffer cell loss during bacterial infection. Immunity. 2015;42(1):10–12. doi:10.1016/j.immuni.2014.12.032.

[81] Sharma J, Li Q, Mishra BB, et al. Lethal pulmonary infection with *Francisella novicida* is associated with severe sepsis. J Leukoc Biol. 2009;86(3):491–504. doi:10.1189/jlb.1208728.

[82] Parmely MJ, Fischer JL, Pinson DM. Programmed cell death and the pathogenesis of tissue injury induced by type A *Francisella tularensis*. FEMS Microbiol Lett. 2009;301(1):1–11. doi:10.1111/j.1574-6968.2009.01791.x.

[83] Rennert K, Otto P, Funke H, et al. A human macrophage – hepatocyte coculture model for comparative studiesof infection and replication of *Francisella tularensis* LVS strain and subspecies holarctica and mediasiatica. BMC Microbiol. 2016;16:2. doi:10.1186/s12866-015-0621-3.

[84] Ganem D, Prince AM. Hepatitis B virus infection-natural history and clinical consequences. N Engl J Med. 2004;350(11):1118–1129. doi:10.1056/NEJMra031087.

[85] Lang PA, Recher M, Honke N, et al. Tissue macrophages suppress viral replication and prevent severe immunopathology in an interferon-I- dependent manner in mice. Hepatology. 2010;52(1):25–32. doi:10.1002/hep.23640.

[86] Cervantes-Barragan L, Kalinke U, Zust R, et al. Type I IFN-mediated protection of macrophages and dendritic cells secures control of murine coronavirus infection. J Immunol. 2009;182(2):1099–1106. doi:10.4049/ jimmunol.182.2.1099.

[87] Raveh D, Kruskal BA, Farland J, et al. T(h)1 and T(h)2 cytokines cooperate to stimulate mannose-receptor-mediated phagocytosis. J Leukocyte Biol. 1998;64(1):108–113.

[88] Lang KS, Lang PA. Balancing viral replication in spleen and liver determines the outcome of systemic virus infection. Z Gastroenterol. 2015;53(12):1432–1435. doi:10.1055/s-0041-109631.

[89] Wilsson A, Lind S, Ohman L, et al. Apoptotic neutrophils containing *Staphylococcus epidermidis* stimulate macrophages to release the proinflammatory cytokines tumor necrosis factor-alpha and interleukin-6. FEMS Immunol Med Microbiol. 2008;53(1):126–135. doi:10.1111/j.1574-695X.2008.00412.x.

[90] Movita D, van de Garde MDB, Biesta P, et al. Inflammatory monocytes recruited to the liver within 24 hours after virus-induced inflammation resemble Kupffer cells but are functionally distinct. J Virol. 2015;89(9):4809–4817. doi:10.1128/JVI.03733-14. Epub 11 Feb 2015.

[91] Hösel M, Quasdorff M, Wiegmann K, et al. Not interferon, but interleukin-6 controls early gene expression in hepatitis B virus infection. Hepatology. 2009;50(6):1773–1782. doi:10.1002/hep.23226.

[92] Boltjes A, van Montfoort N, Biesta PJ, et al. Kupffer cells interact with hepatitis B surface antigen in vivo and in vitro, leading to proinflammatory cytokine production and natural killer cell function. J Infect Dis. 2015;211(8):1268–1278. doi:10.1093/infdis/jiu599.

[93] Li H, Zheng HW, Chen H, et al. Hepatitis B virus particles preferably induce Kupffer cells to produce TGF-β1 over pro-inflammatory cytokines. Dig Liver Dis. 2012;44(4):328–333. doi:10.1016/j.dld.2011.11.005.

[94] Zannetti C, Roblot G, Charrier E, et al. Characterization of the inflammasome in human Kupffer cells in response to synthetic agonists and pathogens. J Immunol. 2016;197(1):356–367. doi:10.4049/jimmunol.1502301.

[95] Jo J, Tan AT, Ussher JE, et al. Toll-like receptor 8 agonist and bacteria trigger potent activation of innate immune cells in human liver. PLoS Pathog. 2014;10:e1004210. doi:10.1371/journal.ppat.1004210.

[96] Ogata H, Chinen T, Yoshida T, et al. Loss of SOCS3 in the liver pro-motes fibrosis by enhancing STAT3-mediated TGF-beta1 production. Oncogene. 2006;25(17):2520–2530. doi:10.1038/sj.onc.1209281.

[97] Liu RM, Gaston PKA. Oxidative stress and glutathione in TGF-beta-mediated fibrogenesis. Free Radic Biol Med. 2010;48(1):1–15. doi:10.1016/j.freeradbiomed.2009.09.026.

[98] Hou X, Hao X, Zheng M, et al. CD205-TLR9-IL-12 axis contributes to CpG-induced oversensitive liver injury in HBsAg transgenic mice by promoting the interaction of NKT cells with Kupffer cells. Cell Mol Immunol. 2016;13:1–10. doi:10.1038/cmi.2015.111.

[99] Li S, Vriend LE, Nasser IA, et al. 2012. Hepatitis C virus-specific t-cell-derived transforming growth factor beta is associated with slow hepatic fibrogenesis. Hepatology. 2012;56(6):2094–2105. doi:10.1002/hep.25951.

[100] Wan YY, Flavell RA. 'Yin-Yang' functions of transforming growth factor-beta and T regulatory cells in immune regulation. Immunol Rev. 2007;220:199–213. doi:10.1111/j.1600-065X.2007.00565.x.

[101] Jee MH, Hong KY, Park JH, et al. New mechanism of hepatic fibrogenesis: hepatitis C virus infection induces transforming growth factor β1 production through glucose-regulated protein 94. J Virol. 2015;90(6):3044–3055. doi:10.1128/JVI.02976-15.

[102] Soota K, Maliakkal B. Ribavirin induced hemolysis: a novel mechanism of action against chronic hepatitis C virus infection. World J Gastroenterol. 2014;20(43):16184–16190. doi:10.3748/wjg.v20.i43.16184.

[103] Crispe IN. Liver antigen-presenting cells. J Hepatol. 2011;54:357–365. doi:10.1016/j.jhep.2010.10.005.

[104] Schlosser J, Eiden M, Vina-Rodriguez A, et al. Natural and experimental hepatitis E virus genotype 3 - infection in European wild boar is transmissible to domestic pigs. Vet Res. 2014;45:121. doi:10.1186/s13567-014-0121-8.

[105] van Egmond M, van Garderen E, van Spriel AB, et al. FcalphaRI-positive liver Kupffer cells: reappraisal of the function of immuno- globulin A in immunity. Nat Med. 2006;6(6):680–685. doi:10.1038/76261.

[106] Canbay A, Feldstein AE, Higuchi H, et al. Kupffer cell engulfment of apoptotic bodies stimulates death ligand and cytokine expression. Hepatology. 2003;38(5):1188–1198. doi:10.1053/jhep.2003.50472.

[107] Brunetti E, White AC Jr. Cestode infestations: hydatid disease and cysticercosis. Infect Dis Clin North Am. 2012;26(2):421–435. doi:10.1016/j.idc.2012.02.001.

[108] Hsu TL, Lin G, Koizumi A, et al. The surface carbohydrates of the *Echinococcus granulosus* larva interact selectively with the rodent Kupffer cell receptor. Mol Biochem Parasitol. 2013;192(1–2):55–59. doi:10.1016/j.molbiopara.2013.12.001.

[109] Díaz A, Casaravilla C, Allen JE, et al. Understanding the laminated layer of larval Echinococcus II: immunology. Trends Parasitol. 2011;27(6):264–273. doi:10.1016/j.pt.2011.01.008.

[110] Díaz A, Casaravilla C, Irigoín F, et al. Understanding the laminated layer of larval Echinococcus I: structure. Trends Parasitol. 2011;27(5):204–213. doi:10.1016/j.pt.2010.12.012.

[111] Díaz A, Fernández C, Pittini A, et al. The laminated layer: recent advances and insights into Echinococcus biology and evolution. Exp Parasitol. 2015;158:23–30. doi: 10.1016/j.exppara.2015.03.019.

[112] Helk E, Bernin H, Ernst T, et al. TNFalpha-mediated liver destruction by Kupffer cells and Ly6Chi monocytes during *Entamoeba histolytica* infection. PLoS Pathog. 2013;9:e1003096. doi:10.1371/journal.ppat.1003096.

[113] Tavares J, Formaglio P, Thiberge S, et al. Role of host cell traversal by the malaria sporozoite during liver infection. 2013;210(5):905–915. doi:10.1084/jem.20121130.

[114] Baer K, Roosevelt M, Clarkson AB Jr, et al. Kupffer cells are obligatory for *Plasmodium yoelii* sporozoite infection of the liver. Cell Microbiol. 2007;9(2):397–412. doi:10.1111/j.1462-5822.2006.00798.x.

[115] McElrath MJ, Murray HW, Cohn ZA. The dynamics of granuloma formation in experimental visceral leishmaniasis. J Exp Med. 1988;167:1927–1937.

[116] Mota MM, Hafalla JCR, Rodriguez A. Migration through host cells activates Plasmodium sporozoites for infection. Nat Med. 2002;8(11):1318–1322. doi:10.1038/nm785.

[117] Goncalves LA, Rodrigues-Duarte L, Rodo J, Vieira de Moraes L, et al. TREM2 governs Kupffer cell activation and explains belr1 genetic resistance to malaria liver stage infection. Proc Natl Acad Sci USA. 2013;110(48):19531–19536. doi:10.1073/pnas.1306873110.

[118] Sturm A, Amino R, van de Sand C, et al. Manipulation of host hepatocytes by the malaria parasite for delivery into liver sinusoids. Science. 2006;313(5791):1287–1290. doi:10.1126/science.1129720.

[119] Lanthier N. Molendi-Coste O, Horsmans Y, et al. Kupffer cell activation is a causal factor for hepatic insulin resistance. Am J Physiol Gastrointest Liver Physiol. 2010;298(1):G107–G116. doi:10.1152/ajpgi.00391.2009.

[120] Lanthier N, Leclercq IA. Liver and systemic insulin resistance. Hepatology. 2014;60:1113–1114. doi:10.1002/hep.27017.

[121] Pais R, Charlotte F, Fedchuk L, et al. A systematic review of follow-up biopsies reveals disease progression in patients with non-alcoholic fatty liver. J Hepatol. 2013;59(3):550–556. doi:10.1016/j.jhep.2013.04.027.

[122] Bertola A, Bonnafous S, Anty R, et al. Hepatic expression patterns of inflammatory and immune response genes associated with obesity and NASH in morbidly obese patients. PLoS One. 2010;5:e13577. doi:10.1371/journal.pone.0013577.

[123] Ganz M, Szabo G. Immune and inflammatory pathways in NASH. Hepatol Int. 2013;7(Suppl 2): 771–781. doi:10.1007/s12072-013-9468-6.

[124] Baeck C, Wei X, Bartneck M, et al. Pharmacological inhibition of the chemokine C-C motif chemokine ligand 2 (monocyte chemoattractant protein 1) accelerates liver fibrosis regression by suppressing Ly-6C(+) macrophage infiltration in mice. Hepatology. 2014;59(3):1060–1072. doi:10.1002/hep.26783.

[125] Mueller JL, Feeney ER, Zheng H, et al. Circulating soluble CD163 is associated with steatohepatitis and advanced fibrosis in nonalcoholic fatty liver disease. Clin Transl Gastroenterol. 2015;6:e114. doi:10.1038/ctg.2015.36.

[126] Imajo K, Fujita K, Yoneda M, et al. Hyperresponsivity to low- dose endotoxin during progression to nonalcoholic steatohepatitis is regulated by leptin-mediated signaling. Cell Metab. 2012;16(1):44–54. doi:10.1016/j.cmet.2012.05.012.

[127] Ye D, Li FY, Lam KS, et al. Toll-like receptor-4 mediates obesity-induced non-alcoholic steatohepatitis through activation of X-box binding protein-1 in mice. Gut. 2012;61(7):1058–1067. doi:10.1136/gutjnl-2011-300269.

[128] Lanthier N, Molendi-Coste O, Cani PD, et al. Kupffer cell depletion prevents but has no therapeutic effect on metabolic and inflammatory changes induced by a high-fat diet. FASEB J. 2011;25(12):4301–4311. doi:10.1096/fj.11-189472.

[129] Tosello-Trampont AC, Landes SG, Nguyen V, et al. Kuppfer cells trigger nonalcoholic steatohepatitis development in diet-induced mouse model through tumor necrosis factor-alpha production. J Biol Chem. 2012;287(48):40161–40172. doi:10.1074/jbc.M112.417014.

[130] McClain C, Barve S, Joshi-Barve S, et al. Dysregulated cytokine metabolism, altered hepatic methionine metabolism and proteasome dysfunction in alcoholic liver disease. Alcohol Clin Exp Res. 2005;29(11-Suppl):180S–188S. doi:10.1097/01.alc.0000189276.34230.f5.

[131] Wan J, Benkdane M, Teixeira-Clerc F, et al. M2 Kupffer cells promote M1 Kupffer cell apoptosis: a protective mechanism against alcoholic and non-alcoholic fatty liver disease. Hepatology. 2014;59(1):130–142. doi:10.1002/hep.26607.

[132] Nath B, Szabo G. Alcohol-induced modulation of signaling pathways in liver parenchymal and nonparenchymal cells: implications for immunity. Semin Liver Dis. 2009;29(2):166–177. doi:10.1055/s-0029-1214372.

[133] Hernandez-Gea V, Friedman SL. Pathogenesis of liver fibrosis. Annu Rev Pathol. 2011;28:425–456. doi:10.1146/annurev-pathol-011110-130246.

[134] Liu C, Tao Q, Sun M, et al. Kupffer cells are associated with apoptosis, inflammation and fibrotic effects in hepatic fibrosis in rats. Lab Invest. 2010;90(12):1805–1816. doi:10.1038/labinvest.2010.123.

[135] Pradere JP, Kluwe J, De MS, et al. Hepatic macrophages but not dendritic cells contribute to liver fibrosis by promoting the survival of activated hepatic stellate cells in mice. Hepatology. 2013;58(4):1461–1473. doi:10.1002/hep.26429.

[136] Baeck C, Wehr A, Karlmark KR, et al. Pharmacological inhibition of the chemokine CCL2 (MCP-1) diminishes liver macrophage infiltration and steatohepatitis in chronic hepatic injury. Gut. 2012;61(3):416–426. doi:10.1136/gutjnl-2011-300304.

[137] Irvine KM, Skoien R, Bokil NJ, et al. Senescent human hepatocytes express a unique secretory phenotype and promote macrophage migration. World J Gastroenterol. 2014;20(47):17851–17862. doi:10.3748/wjg.v20.i47.17851.

[138] Shen H, Sheng L, Chen Z, et al. Mouse hepatocyte over- expression of NF-kappaB-inducing kinase (NIK) triggers fatal macrophage- dependent liver injury and fibrosis. Hepatology. 2014;60:2065–2076. doi:10.1002/hep.27348.

[139] Aoyama T, Inokuchi S, Brenner DA, Seki E. CX3CL1-CX3CR1 interaction pre- vents carbon tetrachloride-induced liver inflammation and fibrosis in mice. Hepatology. 2010;52(4):1390–1400. doi:10.1002/hep.23795.

[140] Gao B. Hepatoprotective and anti-inflammatory cytokines in alcoholic liver disease. J Gastroenterol Hepatol. 2012;27(Suppl 2):89–93. doi:10.1111/j.1440-1746.2011.07003.x.

[141] de Araújo Júnior RF, Garcia VB, de Carvalho Leitão RF, et al. Improves inflammatory response, oxidative stress and fibrosis in the alcohol-induced liver injury in rats by regulating Kuppfer cells and hepatic stellate cells. PLoS One. 2016;11(2):e0148868. doi:10.1371/journal.pone.0148868.

[142] Shen Z, Liu Y, Dewidar B, et al. Delta-like ligand 4 modulates liver damage by down-regulating chemokine expression. Am J Pathol. 2016;6(7):1874–1889. doi:10.1016/j.ajpath.2016.03.010.

[143] Imamura M, Ogawa T, Sasaguri Y, et al. Suppression of macrophage infiltration inhibits activation of hepatic stellate cells and liver fibrogenesis in rats. Gastroenterology. 2005;128(1):138–146. doi: http://dx.doi.org/10.1053/j.gastro.2004.10.005.

[144] Shi J, Shao W, Yang D, et al. Hydrodynamics-based transfection of plasmid encoding receptor activator for nuclear factor kappa B-Fc protects against hepatic ischemia/reperfusion injury in mice. Liver Transpl. 2010;16(5):611–620. doi:10.1002/lt.22030.

[145] Monson KM, Dowlatshahi S, Crockett ET. CXC-chemokine regulation and neutrophil trafficking in hepatic ischemia-reperfusion injury in P-selectin/ICAM-1 deficient mice. J Inflamm. 2007;4:11. doi:10.1186/1476-9255-4-11.

[146] Abu-Amara M, Yang SY, Tapuria N, et al. Liver ischemia/reperfusion injury: processes in inflammatory networks-a review. Liver Transpl. 2010;16(9):1016–1032. doi:10.1002/lt.22117.

[147] Zhang J, Xu P, Song P, et al. CCL2-CCR2 signaling promotes hepatic ischemia/reperfusion. Injury J Surg Res. 2016;202(2):352–362. doi:10.1016/j.jss.2016.02.029.

[148] Palladini G, Ferrigno A, Richelmi P, et al. Role of matrix metalloproteinases in cholestasis and hepatic ischemia/reperfusion injury: a review. World J Gastroenterol. 2015;21(42):12114–12124. doi:10.3748/wjg.v21.i42.12114.

[149] Nakano Y, Kondo T, Matsuo R, et al. Platelet dynamics in the early phase of postischemic liver in vivo. J Surg Res. 2008;149(2):192–198. doi:10.1016/j.jss.2007.09.016.

[150] Luan X, Liu Y, Li M. The role of CD14 and toll-like receptor 4 of Kupffer cells in hepatic ischemia-reperfusion injury in rats. Transpl Proc. 2012;44(4):937–941. doi:10.1016/j.transproceed.2011.11.001.

[151] Gao J, Jiang Z, Wang S, et al. Endoplasmic reticulum stress of Kupffer cells involved in the conversion of natural regulatory T cells to Th17 cells in liver ischemia-reperfusion injury. J Gastroenterol Hepatol. 2016;31(4):883–889. doi:10.1111/jgh.13163.

[152] Ogiku M, Kono H, Hara M, et al. Glycyrrhizin prevents liver injury by inhibition of high-mobility group box 1 production by Kupffer cells after ischemia-reperfusion in rats. J Pharmacol Exp Ther. 2011;339(1):93–98. doi:10.1124/jpet.111.182592.

[153] Arumugam S, Chitteti R, Ramachandran M, et al. TNF-α suppression by glutathione preconditioning attenuates hepatic ischemia reperfusion injury in young and aged rats. Inflamm Res. 2015;64(1):71–81. doi:10.1007/s00011-014-0785-6.

[154] Ouzounidis N, Giakoustidis A, Poutahidis T, et al. Interleukin 18 binding protein ameliorates ischemia/reperfusion-induced hepatic injury in mice. Liver Transpl. 2016;22(2):237–246. doi:10.1002/lt.24359.

[155] Ellett JD, Atkinson C, Evans ZP, et al. Murine Kupffer cells are protective in total hepatic ischemia/reperfusion injury with bowel congestion through IL-10. J Immunol. 2010;184(10):5849–5858. doi:10.4049/jimmunol.0902024.

[156] Meijer C, Wiezer MJ, Diehl AM, et al. Kupffer cell depletion by CI2MDP-liposomes alters hepatic cytokine expression and delays liver regeneration after partial hepatectomy. Liver. 2000;20(1):66–77. doi:10.1034/j.1600-0676.2000.020001066.

[157] Sutter AG, Palanisamy AP, Ellet JD, et al. Intereukin-10 and Kupffer cells protect steatotic mice livers from ischemia-reperfusion injury. Eur Cytokine Netw. 2014;25(4):69–76. doi:10.1684/ecn.2015.0359.

[158] Waller HL, Harper SJ, Hosgood SA, et al. Differential expression of cytoprotective and apoptotic genes in an ischaemia-reperfusion isolated organ perfusion model of the transplanted kidney. Transpl. Int. 2007;20(7):625–631. doi:10.1111/j.1432-2277.2007.00489.x.

[159] Wang C-F, Wang Z-Y, Tao S-F, et al. Preconditioning donor liver with Nodosin perfusion lessens rat ischemia reperfusion injury via heme oxygenase-1 upregulation. J Gastroenterol Hepatol. 2012;27(4):832–840. doi:10.1111/j.1440-1746.2011.06966.x.

[160] Wang Y, Singh R, Lefkowitch JH, et al. Tumor necrosis factor-induced toxic liver injury results from JNK2-dependent activation of caspase-8 and the mitochondrial death pathway. J Biol Chem. 2006;281(22):15258–15267. doi:10.1074/jbc.M512953200.

[161] Lee L-Y, Kaizu T, Toyokawa H, et al. Carbon monoxide induces hypothermia tolerance in Kupffer cells and attenuates liver ischemia/reperfusion injury in rats. Liver Transpl. 2011;17(12):1457–1466. doi:10.1002/lt.22415.

[162] Stienstra R, Saudale F, Duval C, et al. Kupffer cells promote hepatic steatosis via interleukin-1beta-dependent suppression of peroxisome proliferator-activated receptor alpha activity. Hepatology. 2010;51(2):511–522. doi:10.1002/hep.23337.

[163] Endo K, Hori T, Jobara K, et al. Pretransplant replacement of donor liver grafts with recipient Kupffer cells attenuates liver graft rejection in rats. J Gastroenterol Hepatol. 2015;30(5):944–951. doi:10.1111/jgh.12872.

[164] Li T, Zhu J-Y, Wang F-S, et al.Down-regulation of donor Kupffer cell B7 expression reduced recipient lymphocyte activation and secretion of interleukin-2 in vitro. Transpl Proc. 2015;47(10):2985–2990. doi:10.1016/j.transproceed.2015.10.038.

[165] Chen Y, Liang S, Long F, et al. Augmenter of liver regeneration attenuates acute rejection after rat liver transplantation. Am J Surg. 2016;212(1):128–137. doi:10.1016/j.amjsurg.2015.10.036.

[166] Wang B, Zhang Q, Zhu B, et al. Protective effect of gadolinium chloride on early warm ischemia/reperfusion injury in rat bile duct during liver transplantation. PLoS One. 2013;8(1):e52743. doi:10.1371/journal.pone.0052743.

[167] Guermonprez P, Valladeau J, Zitvogel L, et al. Antigen presentation and T cell stimulation by dendritic cells. Annu Rev Immunol. 2002;20:621–667. doi:10.1146/annurev.immunol.20.100301.064828.

[168] Swiecki M, Colonna M. The multifaceted biology of plasmacytoid dendritic cells. Nat Rev Immunol. 2015;15(8): 471–485. doi:10.1038/nri3865.

[169] Gordon S. Alternative activation of macrophages. Nat Rev Immunol. 2003;3:23–35. doi:10.1038/nri978.

[170] Wu K, Kryczek I, Chen L, et al. Kupffer cell suppression of CD8+ T cells in human hepatocellular carcinoma is mediated by B7-H1/ programmed death-1 interactions. Cancer Res. 2009;69(20):8067–8075. doi:10.1158/0008-5472.CAN-09-0901.

[171] Zhang M, Xu S, Han Y, et al. Apoptotic cells attenuate fulminant hepatitis by priming Kupffer cells to produce interleukin-10 through membrane- bound TGF-β. Hepatology. 2011;53(1) 306–316. doi:10.1002/hep.24029.

[172] You Y, Zhang J, Gong J, et al. Mesenchymal stromal cell-dependent reprogramming of Kupffer cells is mediated by TNF-α and PGE2 and is crucial for liver transplant tolerance. Immunol Res. 2015;62(3):292–305. doi: 10.1007/s12026-015-8660-2.

[173] Yan ML, Wang YD, Tian YF, et al. Inhibition of allogeneic T-cell response by Kupffer cells expressing indoleamine 2,3-dioxygenase. World J Gastroenterol. 2010;16(5):636–640. doi:10.3748/wjg.v16.i5.636.

[174] Luan X, Liao W, Lai X, et al. Dynamic changes of indoleamine 2,3-dioxygenase of Kupffer cells in rat liver transplant rejection and tolerance. Transpl Proc. 2012 ;44(4):1045–1047. doi:10.1016/j.transproceed.2012.01.033.

[175] Callery MP, Mangino MJ, Flye MW. Arginine-specific suppression of mixed lymphocyte culture reactivity by Kupffer cells e a basis of portal venous tolerance. Transplant ation.1991;51:1076–1080.

[176] He F, Chen Z, Xu S, et al. Increased CD4+CD25+Foxp3+ regulatory T cells in tolerance induced by portal venous injection. Surgery. 2009;145(6):663–674. doi:10.1016/j.surg.2009.01.016.

[177] Fu W, Zhu J, Qiu Y, et al. Induction of CD4+CD25+T cells and control of cardiac allograft rejection by CD40/CD40L costimulatory pathway blockade in mice. Transpl Proc. 2013;45(2):611–617. doi:10.1016/j.transproceed.2012.10.044.

[178] Jung K, Kang M, Park C, et al. Protective role of V-set and immunoglobulin domain-containing 4 expressed on Kupffer cells during immune-mediated liver injury by inducing tolerance of liver T- and natural killer t-cells. Hepatology. 2012;56(5):1838–1848. doi:10.1002/hep.25906.

[179] Cattley RC, DeLuca J, Elcombe C, et al. Do peroxisome proliferating compounds pose a hepatocarcinogenic hazard to humans? Regul Toxicol Pharmacol. 1998; 27(1):47–60.

[180] Kolios G, Valatas V, Kouroumalis E. Role of Kupffer cells in the pathogenesis of liver disease. World J Gastroenterol. 2006;12(46):7413–7420. doi: 10.3748/wjg.v12.i46.7413.

[181] Wu J, Li J, Salcedo R, et al. The proinflammatory myeloid cell receptor TREM-1 controls Kupffer cell activation and development of hepatocellular car- cinoma. Cancer Res. 2012;72(16):3977–3986. doi:10.1158/0008-5472.CAN-12-0938.

[182] Ehling J, Tacke F. Role of chemokine pathways in hepatobiliary cancer. Cancer Lett. 2016;379(2):173–183. doi:10.1016/j.canlet.2015.06.017.

[183] Li XY, Wu L, Li SW, et al. Effect of CD16a, the surface receptor of Kupffer cells, on the growth of hepatocellular carcinoma cells. Int J Mol Med. 2016;37(6):1465–1474. doi:10.3892/ijmm.2016.2561.

[184] Piccioni F, Fiore E, Bayo J, et al. 4-methylumbelliferone inhibits hepatocellular carcinoma growth by decreasing IL-6 production and angiogenesis. Glycobiology. 2015 ;25(8):825–835. doi:10.1093/glycob/cwv023.

[185] Wilson CL, Jurk D, Fullard N, et al. NF[kappa]B1 is a suppressor of neutrophil-driven hepatocellular carcinoma. Nat Commun. 2015;6:6818. doi:10.1038/ncomms7818.

[186] Koh MY, Gagea M, Sargis T, et al. A new HIF-1α/RANTES driven pathway to hepatocellular carcinoma mediated by germline haploinsufficiency of SART1/HAF Hepatology. 2016;63(5):1576–1591. doi:10.1002/hep.28468.

[187] Van den Eynden GG, Majeed AW, Illemann M, et al. The multifaceted role of the microenvironment in liver metastasis: biology and clinical implications. Cancer Res. 2013;73(7):2031–2043. doi:10.1158/0008-5472.CAN-12-3931.

[188] Palermo NY, Thomas P, Murphy RF, et al. Hexapeptide fragment of carcinoembryonic antigen which acts as an agonist of heterogeneous ribonucleoprotein. J Pept Sci. 2012;18(4):252–260. doi:10.1002/psc.2393.

[189] Ukawa M, Fujiwara Y, Ando H, et al. Hepatic tumor metastases cause enhanced PEGylated liposome uptake by Kupffer cells. Biol Pharm Bull. 2016;39(2):215–220. doi:10.1248/bpb.b15-00611.

[190] Zhang Y, Wang X-F. A niche role for cancer exosomes in metastasis. Nat Cell Biol. 2015;17(6):709–711. doi:10.1038/ncb3181.

[191] Ilkovitch D, Lopez DM. The liver is a site for tumor-induced myeloid-derived suppressor cell accumulation and immunosuppression. Cancer Res. 2009;69(13):5514–5521. doi:10.1158/0008-5472.CAN-08-4625.

[192] Copple BL, Bai S, Moon JO. Hypoxia-inducible factor-dependent production of profibrotic mediators by hypoxic Kupffer cells. Hepatol Res. 2010;40(5):530–539. doi:10.1111/j.1872-034X.2010.00635.x.

[193] Auguste P, Fallavollita L, Wang N, et al. The host inflammatory response promotes liver metastasis by increasing tumor cell arrest and extravasation. Am J Pathol. 2007;170(5):1781–1792.doi:10.2353/ajpath.2007.060886.

[194] Seki S, Nakashima H, Nakashima M, Kinoshita M. Antitumor immunity produced by the liver Kupffer cells, NK cells, NKT cells, and CD8+ CD122+ T cells. Clin Dev Immunol. 2011;2011:868345. doi:10.1155/2011/868345.

[195] Lau WY, Chen GG, Lai PB, et al. Induction of Fas and Fas ligand expression on malignant glioma cells by Kupffer cells, a potential pathway of antiliver metastases. J Surg Res. 2001;101(1):44–51. doi:10.1006/jsre.2001.6253.

Chapter 4

The Role of Monocytes/Macrophages in HBV and HCV Infection

Haijun Li and Zhengkun Tu

Additional information is available at the end of the chapter

http://dx.doi.org/10.5772/intechopen.68353

Abstract

Monocytes/macrophages constitute the first line of defence for external intrusion or infection. Circulatory monocytes represent about 10% of leukocytes in human blood and resident macrophages are distributed in a variety of tissues and organs to maintain body homeostasis. But relatively little is known about the consequences of chronic viral infections on monocytes. Hepatitis B virus (HBV) and Hepatitis C virus (HCV) infections are the most important causes of chronic liver diseases, which may develop to serious and fatal liver pathology, including liver cirrhosis and hepatocellular carcinoma. Whether HBV and HCV infections are cleared or persist is determined by host immune responses. Viral replication takes place inside hepatocytes as soon as infection begins. The secretion of infectious virions or virus proteins can persist for decades at high rates. Chronic infections with HBV and HCV are the result of ineffective anti-viral immune response towards the virus. Interacting with virions or virus proteins, monocytes/macrophages play an important function in the disease process. The role of monocytes/macrophages in HBV and HCV infections or co-infections is discussed in this chapter.

Keywords: monocytes, macrophages, hepatitis B virus, hepatitis C virus

1. Introduction

The significance of the innate immune response as a defence against microbial infections and its link to the adaptive immune responses have become increasingly recognized during the past few years. The activation of the innate immune response generally leads to the production of type I IFNs. Monocytes/macrophages constitute the first line of defence for external intrusion or infection. Circulatory monocytes represent about 10% of leukocytes in human blood and resident macrophages are distributed in a variety of tissues and organs to maintain body homeostasis. But relatively little is known about the consequences of chronic viral infections on monocytes.

Hepatitis B virus (HBV) infection is a major health problem that affects around 350 million people worldwide, despite the availability of a prophylactic vaccine [1]. The number of the chronic HBV infection has already beyond 240 million because a great fraction of patients is unable to clear the virus spontaneously, although there remain a lot of patients clearing the HBV virus at the early stage [2]. Up to date, chronically infected patients are at high risk of developing HBV-related diseases such as liver cirrhosis and hepatocellular carcinoma, which account for 600,000 deaths annually [3]. The interaction between the HBV and an affective inadequate immune response could lead a chronicity of HBV infection [4–6]. Viral replication takes place inside hepatocytes as soon as infection begins. The secretion of infectious virions or virus proteins can persist for decades at high rates. HBV DNA, HBeAg and HBsAg can be easily detected in serum consequently. The levels of these clinical marker means HBV DNA,HBsAg for clinical diagnosis levels could fluctuate for a long time and keep sistency, are a reflection of virus duplicate activity and used to define the patients disease stage [5, 6].

Hepatitis C virus infection is considered as the most serious cause of chronic liver disease and hepatocellular carcinoma worldwide in the past 50 years [7, 8]. The mechanisms by which host immune system lose the supervision and clear the virus are poorly understood. When the HCV invades the body, under the stimulation of the viral proteins, the immune system is accurately activated and regulates the balance between inflammatory injury and immune tolerance. The standard treatment with pegylated interferon and ribavirin has limited effectiveness for the most prevalent viral genotypes (1a/1b) in the U.S in the past years, but the direct-acting anti-viral (DAA) treatment could enhance the effectiveness greatly [9]. While the unaffordable cost and the drug resistance also restrict its widespread use. Unlike HBV infection, no vaccine is currently available to prevent the HCV infection, which is a serious problem we must confront. To understand the HCV-host interactions that lead to viral persistence will help vaccine development and new drug design. The exact mechanism by which HBV escapes immunity is still not known. Interacting with virions or virus proteins, monocytes/macrophages play an important function in the disease process. The role of monocytes/macrophages in HBV and HCV infections is discussed in this chapter.

2. Monocytes/macrophages in HBV infection

Monocytes originated in the bone marrow mainly consist of a part of the innate immune system. Being the first immune barrier, monocytes play multiple roles in the immune system [10]. Such roles include: (1) act as a pool of precursor cell, which replenish to resident macrophages and dendritic cells as soon as needed, and (2) in response to signals of cytokines or chemokines, monocytes can be recruited and migrated to the sites of infected tissues quickly and divided/differentiated into local inflammatory macrophages and dendritic cells to trigger an immune response [11]. Whether HBV infection is cleared or persists is determined by host immune responses [7]. Viral replication takes place inside hepatocytes as soon as infection begins. The secretion of infectious virions or virus proteins can persist for decades at high rates. Hepatitis B virus (HBV) DNA, HBeAg and HBsAg can be easily detected in serum consequently. The levels of these clinical marker means HBV DNA, HBsAg for clinical diagnosis could fluctuate for a long time and keep sistency, are a reflection of virus duplicate activity and used to define the patients disease stage [9].

Circulating monocytes represent about 10% of mononuclear cells in human peripheral blood. Although involving in acute inflammation and wound, relatively little is known about the chronic viral infections on monocytes [12]. One research found that the function of monocytes were impaired in HIV and HCV infection, because of the responsiveness of TLRs [13–15], and Toll-like receptor responsiveness of monocytes in chronic HCV infections [14, 15]. Based on the surface of CD14 and CD16 expression, researches divided monocytes into two distinct subpopulations. $CD14^+$ $CD16^+$ monocytes, which occupy 10–20% of total blood monocytes and produces much more pro-inflammatory cytokines by the stimulation of TLRs ligands, such as TNF and IL-1β. The majority of CD14(high)$CD16^-$ (80–90%) monocytes have been reported to produce relatively high IL-10 and weak TNF [16, 17]. Hepatitis B surface Ag (HBsAg), as a main HBV protein, has been reported to suppress the activity of monocytes through binding to the monocytes. The binding to monocytes was enhanced by a heat-labile serum protein that was inhibited by Ca_2M/Mg_2M, low pH and an HBsAg-specific monoclonal antibody [18]. Hepatitis B surface Ag (HBsAg) inhibits monocytes inflammatory response by means of COX-2 dependence and may regulate natural killer (NK) cell function interfering IFN-γ production by inhibiting IL-18 and IL-12 production [19]. Hepatitis B surface Ag (HBsAg) is the most abundant HBV protein in the liver and in the peripheral blood of chronic hepatitis B (CHB) patients, which can accumulate up to 100 mg/mL in the peripheral blood, and typically outnumbers infectious virions by 1000:1 to 10,000:1 [20]. The high concentration of HBsAg in the blood stream of CHB patients could theoretically contribute to the hampered immune response. Several studies have shown that HBsAg can suppress the release of LPS-induced cytokines in human monocytes by interfering with the TLR signal pathway [21]. These results suggest that HBsAg could be consumed in the macrophages or Kupffer cells (KCs) (shown in **Figure 1**) and alter the innate immune response, which may contribute to the establishment of chronic infections.

Monocyte subset frequencies are altered depending on the clinical phase of the chronic HBV infection [23]. Moreover, HBeAg also plays a regulating action in the HBV infection.

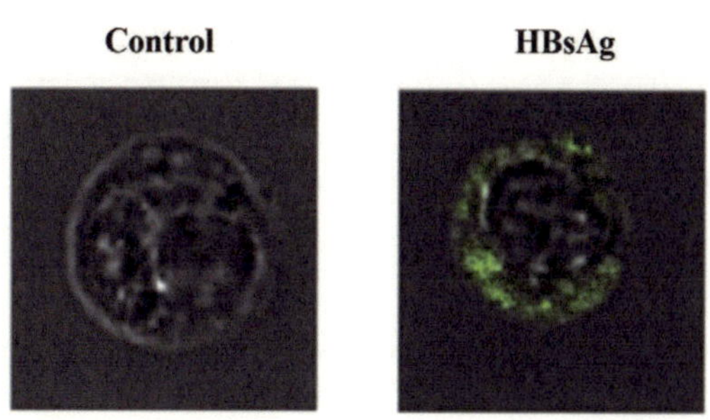

Figure 1. KCs uptake of HBsAg (green) *in vitro* imaged by confocal microscopy [22].

Expression of TLR2 correlates with HBeAg concentration negatively in CHB patients. Stimulation with TLR2 agonists *in vitro* peripheral blood mononuclear cell (PBMC) from HBeAg-positive patients produced less TNF and IL-6 compared to HBeAg-negative patients [24, 25]. Furthermore, exposure of monocytes to HBsAg suppressed LPS-induced TNF and IL-1β production *in vivo* and *in vitro* [26, 27]. Hepatitis B surface Ag (HBsAg) was related to decreased cytokine production induced by the TLR2 ligand (Pam3csk4) in PBMCs from chronic hepatitis B patients *in vivo* [28]. The later research demonstrates that HBsAg selectively inhibits Pam3csk4-stimulated IL-12 production. The mechanism study shows that HBsAg could inhibit JNK-MAPK pathway and provides a mechanism by which HBV evades immunity and maintains its persistence [21].

Kupffer cells (KCs) are the most important innate immune cells in the liver and constitute more than 80% of tissue resident macrophages in the body. Kupffer cells (KCs) account for about 15% of total liver cells, which are more than T cells and liver NK cells. Acting as scavenger cells, KCs remove particulate material from the portal circulation, which has been studied for a long time [29]. Viral infections have been implicated with the KCs in the pathogenesis of inflammatory liver diseases recently [30]. The KCs play an important role in liver injury when the liver is infected by HBV [31].

The liver is continuously exposed to non-pathogenic antigens (from food) and to gut derived lipopolysaccharide (LPS). The LPS is a powerful stimulus for innate immunity through TLR ligation and similarly activates professional antigen-presenting cells (APCs). Kupffer cells modulate the host immune response by the elaboration of IL-10. However, the pro-inflammatory cytokines (IL-12, IL-15 and IL-18) secreted by the Kupffer cells could stimulate NK cell function for secreting IFN-γ [32]. Kupffer cells (KCs) are intravascular macrophages that are continuously exposed to, and tolerant of, bacterial TLR ligands, which are delivered via the portal circulation.

In HBV infection, Kupffer cells participate in many immune responses, including immune cell activation, anti-viral immunity and tissue damage repair [33]. The immune cells cross talk occurs in the infected liver. Kupffer cells regulate T-cell responses by means of the co-stimulatory molecules CD80 and CD86, which are expressed on the cell surface [34]. The ligands of the two molecules on the T cells are CD28 and CTLA-4, respectively. CD86 on APCs stimulates T cells by binding CD28, which occurs before CD80 up expression. CD80 has a higher ability to initiate inhibitory signals through its interaction with CTLA-4 [35–37]. On the other hand, CD80 and CD86 regulate T helper cell differentiation and control adaptive immunity. CD80 mainly drives T-cell differentiation towards a Th1 profile and CD86 leads the differentiation towards a Th2 profile [38–42]. T-cell response in HBV infection mainly initiates Th2 immune response rather than Th1. The production of IL-10 was reported in many researches but the Th1 responses and cytokine production are weak when compared with resolver [43, 44].

Kupffer cells (KCs) and infiltrating monocytes/macrophages are main APCs to regulate adoptive immune response but must avoid hyper-activation of the immune system through expressing inhibitory molecules PD-L1 and PD-L2. The levels of PD-L1 and CD80/CD86 signals on APCs control the magnitude of T-cell activation [45–47]. One study has investigated the expression of CD80 and CD86 on KCs in HBV infection. This study found that only few KCs express these molecules [48]. The different expressions of CD80, CD86 and PD-L1 in KCs in the portal areas of the liver were explored together with the correlation of their expressions with the fibrosis score and grade of inflammation during HBV infection. The HBV virus and the protein function on monocytes/macrophages are listed in **Table 1**.

Virus/protein	Cell receptor	Cell signal	Cytokines
HBsAg	TLR2	MAPK/JNK	IL-12
	TLR4	PI3K	TNF-a, IL-1b
HBeAg	TLR2	C-Jun/JNK	TNF-a, IL-6
HBVcore	TLR2/4	PI3K/JNK	TNF-a, IL-6,IL-12
HBV DNA	TLR7/9	RGI	IL-12, IL-18

Table 1. Monocytes'/macrophages' function in HBV infection.

3. Monocytes/macrophages in HCV infection

Hepatitis C virus (HCV) is also a cause of serious liver diseases as well as other extra hepatic pathologies especially in the developed countries. A classical combination of the drugs pegylated interferon and ribavirin used as standard treatment for decades. Recently, some other drugs have been approved that may enhance the effectiveness to a great extent. These drugs are designed to block the virus duplication by interfering with specific viral proteins. Rational therapies and effective vaccine can be designed if HCV replication is understood totally. Monocytes appeared to contain the core protein of HCV by flow cytometry *in vitro* infected experiment, suggesting that HCV was inside the monocytes [49]. Different types of monocytic cell lineages have been investigated, with $CD14^{+}$, $CD16^{++}$ and $CD14^{++}$, $CD16^{++}$ but not with $CD14^{+}$, $CD16^{-}$ cells being found infected [50]. These studies suggest that different cell types allow replication of slightly different versions of HCV.

Monocytes are not only infected by HCV virions, but also influenced by virus proteins. Chronic activation of monocytes and macrophages is seen in HCV and correlates with liver damage [51, 30]. Monocytes had the highest gal-9 levels in chronically infected HCV patients suggests that they may be a source of T cell inhibitory gal-9 in HCV infection. Toll-like receptors (TLR) have a critical role in innate immunity against pathogens. During chronic HCV infection, interleukin-12 (IL-12) produced by monocytes/macrophages is significantly suppressed. Programmed death-1 (PD-1), an inhibitory receptor on immune cells, plays a pivotal role in suppressing T-cell responses during chronic viral infection. IL-12 production decreased on monocytes/macrophages in HCV infection correlates the up-regulation of PD-1 on cell surface. IL-12 production resumed when PD-1/PD-L1 antibody or IFN/RBV treatment was carried out. The possible mechanism is that the STAT-1 phosphorylation is enhanced during the treatment [52]. Tim-3, acting as a negative regulator, inhibits monocytes'/macrophages' function in HCV infection in some researches [53].

Myeloid-derived suppressor cell (MDSC) is a kind of inhibitory cell that originated in the bone marrow and was first identified as natural suppressor cell in tumour-bearing mice in the mid-1960s [54]. Myeloid-derived suppressor cell (MDSC) originated in the bone marrow and later differentiated/divided into granulocytes, macrophages or mature dendritic cells [55, 56]. Myeloid-derived suppressor cell (MDSC) migrates or accumulates in the tumours, spleen, bone marrow and blood under different pathological conditions. Based on the different cell surface markers and cell origin, the MDSC can be divided into monocyte (Mo), granulocyte and endothelial-committed subsets. Myeloid-derived suppressor cell (MDSC) represents a cell type that suppresses the function of other immune cells and creates a suppressive environment. Studies revealed that MDSC numbers correlate with T-cell frequency inversely in the peripheral blood [57]. T-cell responses can be suppressed by MDSCs through numerous mechanisms [58–60]. In patients with HCV infection, T-cell function is impaired according to the clinical observation. Hepatitis C virus (HCV) core protein and polyI:C induce TNF-α (pro-inflammatory cytokine), IL-10 (immunomodulatory cytokine) and IFN-γ (anti-viral cytokine) secretions from monocytes. Then, monocytes are reprogrammed to acquire or lose the immunosuppressive (MDSC) phenotype through these cytokines. Hepatitis C virus–induced Mo-MDSC production was attributed to the PI3K pathway via induction of IL-10 and TNF-α secretion [61]. The HBV virus and the protein function on monocytes/macrophages are listed in **Table 2**.

Virus/protein	Cell receptor	Cell signal	Cytokines
HCVcore	TLR2	MYD88	IL-6, IL-10
HCV RNA	TLR7/8	CD81	IL-1b, IL-12
HCV dsRNA	TLR3	ISG15/56	IFNα/β
NS3	TLR2	RGI	IL-1b, IL-6, TNF-α

Table 2. Monocytes'/macrophages' function in HCV infection.

4. Monocytes/macrophages in HBV/HCV co-infection

Despite their different replication strategies and life cycles, HBV and HCV have similar modes of transmission through bodily fluid, and both have developed highly successful ways to establish chronic hepatitis [62]. Liver injury and disease progression are thought to be driven by the interaction between viruses and host immune responses in both infections [63–66]. Given their similar modes of transmission, HBV/HCV co-infection occurs frequently in endemic areas although its prevalence is exactly unknown [67]. Between 2 and 10% of anti–HCV-positive patients also test positive for HBsAg, while 5–20% of patients with chronic HBV infection test positive for anti-HCV antibodies [68]. It has been reported that HBV/HCV co-infection leads to more severe liver disease and a higher prevalence of liver cancer than non-infection [69], but an inverse relationship between the replication of each virus within some co-infected patients has been noted [70–74]. Hepatitis B virus-Hepatitis C virus co-infection involves complex viral interaction; HBV and HCV can replicate in the same cells *in vitro* with no evidence of interference between them [75, 76]. Therefore, the viral interference observed in HBV/HCV co-infected patients *in vivo* is probably due to indirect mechanisms mediated by innate and/or adaptive host immune responses.

Hepatitis B virus-Hepatitis C virus co-infection is a blank field because of lack of robust cell and animal experimental model. Our research group attempts to do some basic experiments in HBV-HCV co-infection. Human primary peripheral blood monocytes were cultured for 2 days in increasing concentrations of infectious HCV, infectious HBV or both viruses together. As expected, the HCV, HBV and the two viruses together suppressed the expression of HLA-DR and TRAIL on monocytes, and increased the expression of PD-L1 and the secretion of IL-10, similar to the effects of recombinant HCV. In addition, we also uncovered previously unknown immune suppressive effects in both HCV and HBV, and the two viruses together strongly suppressed the expression of genes encoding stat1 and stat2, thereby disabling IFN signalling. These findings help to explain the well-known propensity of both HCV and HBV to induce T-cell immune suppression and clonal exhaustion, but they do not explain the anti-HCV effect of HBV infection *in vivo*. Other cell types, or cytokines, or both, may be playing a role in association with HBV mediated suppression of HCV.

To identify cytokines that were secreted in response to HBV, but not HCV, we performed experiments in which viruses were titrated either alone, or against a fixed concentration of the other virus, and observed that HBV induced IL-1β and IL-12 secretion, while HCV did not. Furthermore, the presence of HCV did not suppress the induction of either IL-1β or IL-12 by HBV. Since cytokine expression is regulated by a number of genes, we next measured the expression level of the associated genes. We observed novel emergent properties when the two viruses were combined. That is, Nfkb1 was not induced by HBV alone. It was induced by low concentrations of HCV, but then suppressed by higher concentrations. However, with HCV and HBV combined, the expression of this gene was sustained across a wide range of viral titers. Similarly, the Ifr1 gene was not affected by HBV alone but was modestly elevated by HCV, but drastically elevated with HCV and HBV combined. The secretion of TNF-α was strongly induced by HBV, but not by HCV, and modestly suppressed in the presence of both viruses together. Based on experiments in which human blood monocytes were exposed to intact HBV, intact HCV, or both viruses together, our results showed that both viruses exert strong immunosuppressive effects.

5. Perspectives

Our understanding of the role of monocytes/macrophages in HBV or HCV is far from completion. Nevertheless, the anti-viral roles of monocytes/macrophages will be appreciated by binding and/or uptake of virus leading to immune recognition and the production of pro-inflammatory or anti-inflammatory mediators resulting in (1) activation of neighbouring cells, such as NK cells and $CD8^+$ T cells, (2) blockage in viral replication in hepatocytes and (3) attraction, activation and interaction with other immune cells, including ILCs, pDCs and Tregs, which will further increase the anti-viral and inflammatory response. In the early phases after infection, the immune activating roles of monocytes/macrophages are beneficial to help the body cause anti-virus response and clear virus and dead cell. But the situation will turn to the other side if the infection develops into chronic. The strong immune activity may also contribute to tissue damage and the development of fibrosis, cirrhosis and HCC. Furthermore, immune regulatory functions of monocytes/macrophages have been described, which may counteract the development of effective anti-viral immunity and support viral persistence and related disease pathogenesis.

Intrahepatic macrophages become an interesting and complex cellular target for treatment options and hot point in viral hepatitis with the growing appreciation of the roles of intrahepatic macrophages in both protective and harmful responses. With the development of flow and cell sorting technology, identifying phenotypical and/or functional characteristics discriminating KC from infiltrating macrophages will become easy day after day. Despite the existence of a HBV, vaccine is used widely but the already HBV infected population also be at high risk of developing to liver fibrosis and liver cancer. The standard treatment with pegylated interferon and ribavirin has limited effectiveness for the most prevalent viral genotypes (1a/1b) in the U.S in the past years, but the DAA treatment could enhance the effectiveness greatly. Also, the unaffordable price and the drug resistance also restrict its widespread use. Unlike HBV infection, no vaccine is currently available to prevent HCV, which is a serious problem we must confront. To understand the HCV-host interactions that lead to viral persistence will help vaccine development and new drug design. The exact mechanism of monocytes/macrophages in HBV and HCV infection will provide us new insight into and confidence to overcome the virus.

Author details

Haijun Li and Zhengkun Tu*

*Address all correspondence to: tuzhengkun@hotmail.com

Institute of Translational Medicine, The First Hospital, Jilin University, Changchun, China

References

[1] Honer Zu, Siederdissen C, Cornberg M. The role of HBsAg levels in the current management of chronic HBV infection. Ann Gastroenterol, 2014, 27: 105–12.

[2] Ott JJ, Stevens GA, Groeger J, Wiersma ST. Global epidemiology of hepatitis B virus infection: new estimates of age-specific HBsAg seroprevalence and endemicity. Vaccine, 2012, 30: 2212–2219.

[3] Peppa D, Gill US, Reynolds G, Easom NJ, Pallett LJ, Schurich A, et al. Upregulation of a death receptor renders antiviral T cells susceptible to NK cellmediated deletion. J Exp Med, 2013, 210: 99–114.

[4] Boonstra A, Woltman AM, Janssen HL. Immunology of hepatitis B and hepatitis C virus infections. Best Pract Res Clin Gastroenterol, 2008, 22: 1049–1061.

[5] Ganem D, Prince AM. Hepatitis B virus infection-natural history and clinical consequences. N Engl J Med, 2004, 350: 1118–1129.

[6] Rehermann B, Nascimbeni M. Immunology of hepatitis B virus and hepatitis C virus infection. Nat Rev Immunol, 2005, 5: 215–229.

[7] Lauer GM, Walker BD. Hepatitis C virus infection. N Engl J Med, 2001, 345: 41–52.

[8] Dustin LB, Rice CM. Flying under the radar: the immunobiology of hepatitis C. Annu Rev Immunol, 2007, 25: 71–99.

[9] Shepard CW, Finelli L, Alter MJ. Global epidemiology of hepatitis C virusinfection. Lancet Infect Dis, 2005, 5: 558–567.

[10] Artis D, Spits H. The biology of innate lymphoid cells. Nature, 2015, 517(7534): 293–301.

[11] Shi J, Zhao Y, Wang Y, Gao W, Ding J, Li P, Hu L, Shao F. Inflammatory caspases are innate immune receptors for intracellular LPS. Nature, 2014, 514(7521): 187–92.

[12] Dunn C, Peppa D, Khanna P, Nebbia G, Jones M, Brendish N, et al. Temporal analysis of early immune responses in patients with acute hepatitis B virus infection. Gastroenterology, 2009, 137: 1289–300.

[13] Nockher WA, Bergmann L, Scherberich JE. Increased soluble CD14 serum levels and altered CD14 expression of peripheral blood monocytes in HIV-infected patients. Clin Exp Immunol, 1994, 98: 369–374.

[14] Nockher WA, Scherberich JE. Expanded CD14+ CD16+ monocyte subpopulation in patients with acute and chronic infections undergoing hemodialysis. Infect Immun, 1998, 66: 2782–2790.

[15] Liu BS, Groothuismink ZM, Janssen HL, Boonstra A. Role for IL-10 in inducing functional impairment of monocytes upon TLR4 ligation in patients with chronic HCV infections. J Leukoc Biol, 2011, 89: 981–988.

[16] Peng C, Liu BS, de Knegt RJ, Janssen HL, Boonstra A. The response to TLR ligation of human CD16(+)CD14(−) monocytes is weakly modulated as a consequence of persistent infection with the hepatitis C virus. Mol Immunol, 2011, 48: 1505–1511.

[17] Auffray C, Sieweke MH, Geissmann F. Blood monocytes: development, heterogeneity, and relationship with dendritic cells. Annu Rev Immunol, 2009, 27: 669–692.

[18] Gehring AJ, Haniffa M, Kennedy PT, Ho ZZ, Boni C, Shin A, Banu N, Chia A, Lim SG, Ferrari C, Ginhoux F, Bertoletti A. Mobilizing monocytes to cross-present circulating viral antigen in chronic infection. J Clin Invest, 2013, 123(9): 3766–76.

[19] Cheng J, Imanishi H, Morisaki H, Liu W, Nakamura H, Morisaki T, Hada T. Recombinant HBsAg inhibits LPS-induced COX-2 expression and IL-18 production by interfering

with the NFkappaB pathway in a human monocytic cell line, THP-1. J Hepatol, 2005, 43(3): 465–71.

[20] Dammermann W, Bentzien F, Stiel EM, Kühne C, Ullrich S, Schulze Zur Wiesch J, Lüth S. Development of a novel IGRA assay to test T cell responsiveness to HBV antigens in whole blood of chronic Hepatitis B patients. J Transl Med, 2015, 13: 157.

[21] Wang S, Chen Z, Hu C, Qian F, Cheng Y, Wu M, Shi B, Chen J, Hu Y, Yuan Z. Hepatitis B virus surface antigen selectively inhibits TLR2 ligand-induced IL-12 production inmonocytes/macrophages by interfering with JNK activation. J Immunol, 2013, 190(10): 5142–51.

[22] Boltjes A, van Montfoort N,. Biesta PJ, et al. Kupffer cells interact with hepatitis B surface antigen in vivo and in vitro, leading to proinflammatory cytokine production and natural killer cell function. J Infect Dis, 2015, 211: 1268–1278.

[23] Anthony DD, Umbleja T, Aberg JA, Kang M, Medvik K, et al. Lower peripheral blood CD14+monocyte frequency and higher CD34+ progenitor cell frequency are associated with HBV vaccine induced response in HIV infected individuals. Vaccine, 2011, 29: 3558–3563.

[24] Zhang JY, Zou ZS, Huang A, Zhang Z, Fu JL, et al. Hyper-activated proinflammatory CD16 monocytes correlate with the severity of liver injury and fibrosis in patients with chronic hepatitis B. PLoS ONE, 2011, 6: e17484.

[25] Visvanathan K, Skinner NA, Thompson AJV, Riordan SM, Sozzi V, et al. Regulation of Toll-like receptor-2 expression in chronic hepatitis B by the precore protein. Hepatology, 2007, 45: 102–110.

[26] Riordan SM, Skinner N, Kurtovic J, Locarnini S, Visvanathan K. Reduced expression of toll-like receptor 2 on peripheral monocytes inpatients with chronic hepatitis B. Clin Vaccine Immunol, 2006, 13: 972–974.

[27] Boltjes A, Groothuismink ZM, van Oord GW, Janssen HL, Woltman AM, Boonstra A. Monocytes from chronic hbv patients react in vitro to hbsag and tlr by producing cytokines irrespective of stage of disease. PLoS One, 2014, 9(5): e97006.

[28] Chen Z, Cheng Y, Xu Y, Liao J, Zhang X, Hu Y, Zhang Q, Wang J, Zhang Z, Shen F, Yuan Z. Expression profiles and function of Toll-like receptors 2 and 4 in peripheral blood mononuclear cells of chronic hepatitis B patients. Clin Immunol, 2008, 128: 400–408.

[29] Vollmar B, Menger MD. The hepatic microcirculation: mechanistic contributions and therapeutic targets in liver injury and repair. Physiol Rev, 2009, 89: 1269–1339.

[30] Heydtmann M. Macrophages in hepatitis B and hepatitis C virus infections. J Virol, 2009, 83: 2796–2802.

[31] Wu Z, Han M, Chen T, Yan W, Ning Q. Acute liver failure: mechanisms of immune-mediated liver injury. Liver Int, 2010, 30: 782–794.

[32] Tu Z, Pierce RH, Kurtis J, et al. Hepatitis C virus core protein subverts the anti-viral activities of human kupffer cells. Gastroenterology, 2010, 138: 305–314.

[33] Boltjes A, Movita D, Boonstra A, Woltman AM. The role of Kupffer cells in hepatitis B and hepatitis C virus infections. J Hepatol, 2014, 61: 660–671.

[34] Romo-Tena J, Gomez-Martin D, Alcocer-Varela J. CTLA-4 and autoimmunity: new insights into the dual regulator of tolerance. Autoimmun Rev, 2013, 12: 1171–1176.

[35] Manzotti CN, Liu MXP, Burke F, Dussably L, Zheng Y, Sansom DM. Integration of CD28 and CTLA-4 function results in differential responses of T cells to CD80 and CD86. Eur J Immunol, 2006, 36: 1413–1422.

[36] Sansom DM. CD28, CTLA-4 and their ligands: who does what and to whom? Immunology, 2000, 101:169–177.

[37] Zhang Q, Wang HY, Wei F, Liu XB, Paterson JC, Roy D, et al. Cutaneous T cell lymphoma expresses immunosuppressive CD80 (B7-1) cell surface protein in a STAT5-Dependent Manner. J Immunol, 2014, 192: 2913–2919.

[38] Asai-Tajiri Y, Matsumoto K, Fukuyama S, Kan-o K, Nakano T, Tonai K, et al. Small interfering RNA against CD86 during allergen challenge blocks experimental allergic asthma. Respir Res, 2014, 15.

[39] Balkhi MY, Latchumanan VK, Singh B, Sharma P, Natarajan K. Cross-regulation of CD86 byCD80 differentially regulates T helper responses from Mycobacterium tuberculosis secretory antigen activated dendritic cell subsets. J Leukoc Biol, 2004, 75: 874–883.

[40] Maj T, Slawek A, Chelmonska-Soyta A. CD80 and CD86 costimulatory molecules differentially regulate OT-II CD4(+) T lymphocyte proliferation and cytokine response in cocultures with antigen presenting cells derived from pregnant and pseudopregnant mice. Mediators Inflamm, 2014:769239.

[41] Slavik JM, Hutchcroft JE, Bierer BE. CD28/CTLA-4 and CD80/CD86 families—signaling and function. Immunol Res, 1999, 19: 1–24.

[42] Yoshida T, Hachimura S, Ishimori M, Ise W, Totsuka M, Ametani A, et al. Interleukin 12 and CD86 regulate Th1 and Th2 development induced by a range of antigen doses presented by Peyer's patch and spleen cells. Cytotechnology, 2003, 43: 81–88.

[43] Bertoletti A, DElios MM, Boni C, DeCarli M, Zignego AL, Durazzo M, et al. Different cytokine profiles of intrahepatic T cells in chronic hepatitis B and hepatitis C virus infections. Gastroenterology, 1997, 112:193–199.

[44] Chang JJ, Thompson AJV, Visvanathan K, Kent SJ, Cameron PU, Wightman F, et al. The phenotype of hepatitis B virus-specific T cells differ in the liver and blood in chronic hepatitis B virus infection. Hepatology, 2007, 46: 1332–1340.

[45] Cros J, Cagnard N, Woollard K, Patey N, Zhang SY, et al. Human CD14dim monocytes patrol and sense nucleic acids and viruses via TLR7 and TLR8 receptors. Immunity, 2010, 33: 375–386.

[46] Carter LL, Fouser LA, Jussif J, Fitz L, Deng B, Wood CR, et al. PD-1: PD-L inhibitory pathway affects both CD4(+) and CD8(+) T cells and is overcome by IL-2. Eur J Immunol, 2002, 32:634–643.

[47] Trautmann L, Said EA, Halwani R, Janbazian L, Chomont N, El-Far M, et al. Programmed death1: a critical regulator of T-cell function and a strong target for immunotherapies for chronic viral infections. Curr Opin HIV AIDS, 2007, 2: 219–227.

[48] Leifeld L, Trautwein C, Dumoulin FL, Manns MP, Sauerbruch T, Spengler U. Enhanced expression of CD80 (B7-1), CD86 (B7-2), and CD40 and their ligands CD28 and CD154 in fulminant hepatic failure. Am J Pathol, 1999, 154: 1711–1720.

[49] Bouffard P, Hayashi PH, Acevedo R, Levy N, Zeldis JB. Hepatitis C virus is detected in a monocyte/macrophage subpopulation of peripheral blood mononuclear cells of infected patients. J Infect Dis, 1992, 166: 1276–1280.

[50] Coquillard G, Patterson BK. Determination of hepatitis C virus-infected, monocyte lineage reservoirs in individuals with or without HIV coinfection. J Infect Dis, 2009, 200: 947–954.

[51] Dolganiuc A, Norkina O, Kodys K, Catalano D, Bakis G, Marshall C, Mandrekar P, Szabo G. Viral and host factors induce macrophage activation and loss of toll-like receptor tolerance in chronic HCV infection. Gastroenterology, 2007, 133, 1627–1636.

[52] Cheng J Ma,Lei Ni,Ying Zhang, et al. PD-1negatively regulates interleukin-12 expression by limiting STAT-1 phosphorylation in monocytes/macrophages during chronic hepatitis C virus infection. Immunology, 2010, 132: 421–431.

[53] Ying Zhang, Cheng JMa, Jia MWang, et al. Tim-3 negatively regulates IL-12 expression by monocytes in HCV infection. PLoS ONE, 2011, 6(5): e19664.

[54] Lappat EJ, Cawein M, Study of the leukemoid response to transplantable a-280 tumor in mice, Cancer Res, 1964, 24: 302–311.

[55] Bunt SK, Clements VK, Hanson EM, Sinha P, Ostrand-Rosenberg S. Inflammation enhances myeloid-derived suppressor cell cross-talk by signaling through Toll-like receptor 4. J Leukoc Biol, 2009, 85: 996–1004.

[56] Hu CE, Gan J, Zhang RD, Cheng YR, Huang GJ. Up-regulated myeloid-derived suppressor cell contributes to hepatocellular carcinoma development by impairing dendritic cell function. Scand J Gastroenterol, 2011, 46: 156–164.

[57] Donkor MK, Lahue E, Hoke TA, Shafer LR, Coskun U, Solheim JC, Gulen D, Bishay J, Talmadge JE. Mammary tumor heterogeneity in the expansion of myeloid-derived suppressor cells. Int Immunopharmacol, 2009, 9: 937–948.

[58] Poschke I, Mougiakakos D, Hansson J, Masucci GV, Kiessling R. Immature immunosuppressive CD14+HLA-DR-/low cells in melanoma patients are Stat3hi and overexpress CD80, CD83, and DC-sign. Cancer Res, 2010, 70: 4335–4345.

[59] Gabrilovich DI, Nagaraj S. Myeloid-derived suppressor cells as regulators of the immune system. Nat Rev Immunol, 2009, 9: 162–174.

[60] Hoechst B, Ormandy LA, Ballmaier M, Lehner F, Krüger C, Manns MP, Greten TF, Korangy F. A new population of myeloid-derived suppressor cells in hepatocellular carcinoma patients induces CD4(+)CD25(+)Foxp3(+) T cells, Gastroenterology, 2008, 135: 234–243.

[61] Pang X, Song H, Zhang Q, Tu Z, Niu J. Hepatitis C virus regulates the production of monocytic myeloid-derived suppressor cells from peripheral blood mononuclear cells through PI3K pathway and autocrine signaling. Clin Immunol, 2016, 164: 57–64.

[62] Mitchell AE, Colvin HM, Palmer Beasley R. Institute of medicine recommendations for the prevention and control of hepatitis B and C. Hepatology, 2010, 51(3): 729–33.

[63] Rehermann B, Bertoletti A. Immunological aspects of antiviral therapy of chronic hepatitis B virus and hepatitis C virus infections. Hepatology, 2015, 61(2): 712–21.

[64] Yi G, Wen Y, Shu C, Han Q, Konan KV, Li P, Kao CC. Hepatitis C virus NS4B can suppress STING accumulation to evade innate immune responses. J Virol, 2015, 90(1): 254–65.

[65] Park JJ, Wong DK, Wahed AS. HBV-specific and global T-cell dysfunction in chronic hepatitis B. Gastroenterology, 2015, 15: 01736–9.

[66] Pallett LJ, Gill US, Quaglia A. Metabolic regulation of hepatitis B immunopathology by myeloid-derived suppressor cells. Nat Med, 2015, 21(6): 591–600.

[67] Gordon SC, Sherman KE. Treatment of HBV/HCV coinfection: releasing the enemy within. Gastroenterology, 2009, 136(2): 393–6.

[68] Bini EJ, Perumalswami PV. Hepatitis B virus infection among American patients with chronic hepatitis C virus infection: prevalence, racial/ethnic differences, and viral interactions. Hepatology, 2010, 51:759–766.

[69] Cho LY, Yang JJ, Ko KP. Coinfection of hepatitis B and C viruses and risk of hepatocellular carcinoma: systematic review and meta-analysis. Int J Cancer, 2011, 128(1): 176–84.

[70] Bellecave P, Gouttenoire J, Gajer M, et al. Hepatitis B and C virus coinfection: a novel model system reveals the absence of direct viral interference. Hepatology, 2009, 50: 46–55.

[71] Wieland SF, Asabe S, Engle RE, et al. Limited hepatitis B virus replication space in the chronically hepatitis c virus-infected liver. J Virol, 2014, 88(9): 5184–5188.

[72] Liu CJ, Chu YT, Shau WY, et al. Treatment of patients with dual hepatitis C and B by peginterferon α and ribavirin reduced risk of hepatocellular carcinoma and mortality. Gut, 2014, 63(3): 506–14.

[73] Collins JM, Raphael KL, Terry C, et al. Hepatitis B virus reactivation during successful treatment of hepatitis c virus with sofosbuvir and simeprevir. Clin Infect Dis, 2015, 61(8): 1304–6.

[74] Wahle RC, Perez RM, Pereira PF, et al. Hepatitis B virus reactivation after treatment for hepatitis C in hemodialysis patients with HBV/HCV coinfection. Braz J Infect Dis, 2015, 19(5): 533–7.

[75] Bellecave P, Sarasin-Filipowicz M, Donzé O, et al. Tschopp cleavage of mitochondrial antiviral signaling protein in the liver of patients with chronic hepatitis C correlates with a reduced activation of the endogenous interferon system. Hepatology, 2010, 51(4): 1127–36.

[76] Yang D, Zuo C, Wang X, et al. Complete replication of hepatitis B virus and hepatitis C virus in a newly developed hepatoma cell line. PNAS, 2014, 111(13): E1264–73.

Chapter 5

Dendritic Cell Endocytosis Essential for Viruses and Vaccines

Kenneth C. McCullough and Rajni Sharma

Additional information is available at the end of the chapter

http://dx.doi.org/10.5772/67779

Abstract

Protective immune defences are dependent upon critical roles played by dendritic cells (DCs), rendering them important targets for both vaccine delivery and virus infection. Studies in these areas led to successful development of targeted vaccine delivery, including synthetic virus-like particle (SVLP) and nanoparticulate RNA vaccines. A major consideration is DC endocytosis, whereby the different endocytic routes influencing the outcome. Rapid clathrin-mediated endocytosis likely favours degradative pathways. Slower processes such as macropinocytosis, caveolar endocytosis and retrograde transport to endoplasmic reticulum relate more to the processing rates leading to antigen presentation by DCs. These pathways are also influential in promoting the initiation of virus replication following infection. DC endocytosis of RNA viruses and RNA vaccines must lead to cytosolic translocation of the RNA for translation, relating to the process of antigen cross-presentation. One can learn from observations on both virus infections and cross-presentation for delivering RNA vaccines. Accordingly, recent advances in nanoparticulate delivery have been applied with self-amplifying replicon RNA (RepRNA), providing efficient delivery to DCs and promoting replicon-encoded antigen translation. Through realising the important relationships between DC endocytic pathways and induction of immune responses, delivery of SVLP and RepRNA vaccines to DCs offers high value for the development of future synthetic vaccine platforms.

Keywords: dendritic cells, endocytosis, virus infection, vaccines, SVLPs, self-amplifying RNA

1. Introduction

While protective immune defences are reliant upon robust antibody-mediated (B-lymphocyte) and concomitant T-lymphocyte response, their development is dependent on antigen delivery leading to processing and presentation by dendritic cells (DCs), a critical player for robust immune defence development, and therefore efficacious vaccination [1–9]. Induction of antibody (humoral) and cell-mediated immune (CMI) defences requires virus or vaccine interaction with the conventional DC (cDC) subsets, the 'professional antigen presenting cells' [3, 6–12] (**Figure 1**). The manner by which these cDCs handle the antigen derived from an infection or vaccination defines the characteristics of adaptive immune defence development (**Figure 2**). Considering that many pathogen infections induce both humoral and CMI defences, vaccines inducing both arms of immune defence increase the potential for inducing robust immune defences. Accordingly, live attenuated vaccines should more closely mimic pathogen infection and therefore induce immune defence characteristics more related to convalescent immunity.

Understanding the cell biological elements providing DCs with their functionality has been possible from studies on both effective convalescent immunity and that induced by efficacious vaccination. Whether the studies focussed on virus infection or efficacious vaccine delivery, particular routes of endocytosis were observed to dominate. Through this, the power of DCs as the 'professional antigen-presenting cell' was determined [1, 3, 4, 6–8]. Yet, most current vaccines are inactivated or subunit/split vaccines. Being non-replicative, only a limited amount of antigen can be provided, namely that within the vaccine dose, in contrast to the much greater antigen levels produced during infection and from a live vaccine. Such non-replicative vaccines induce more restricted immune defence characteristics, in terms of humoral versus CMI immunity and the robustness (longevity) of that immunity, than observed with convalescent immunity or that induced by a replicating vaccine.

Of course, pathogen infection can induce undesirable clinical symptoms influencing the development of convalescent immune defence, which can be avoided by employing non-pathogenic replicating vaccines. Unfortunately, safe and efficacious live vaccines are not available for the majority of pathogens. Nonetheless, lessons can be learnt from convalescent immunity [9, 13]. A major consideration is the capacity of replicating vaccines to mimic the pathogen infection such as producing several rounds of antigen production, increasing the effective antigen dose, involving different antigen-presentation pathways, promoting different arms of immune responses and thus increasing the efficacy of immune defence induction [9].

Resolution of this situation is showing promise from the more recent application of synthetic biology to create both synthetic virus-like particles (SVLPs) [14–16] and self-amplifying/replicating RNA (replicon or RepRNA) vaccines [9, 13, 17–20], but also from advances in studies on virus infections. It has been observed that the majority of endocytosed material may well traverse rapid clathrin-mediated pathways, which is more likely favouring degradation of the internalised material [9, 21–25] (**Figure 3**, pathway (a)). Slower kinetics of endocytosis would favour the processing required for a particular vaccine to prove efficacious or a virus to initiate its replication. Such outcomes are seen with macropinocytosis and caveolar endocytosis (**Figure 1**; **Figure 3** pathway (b)), as well as endocytosis into sorting endosomes for retrograde

http://dx.doi.org/10.5772/67779

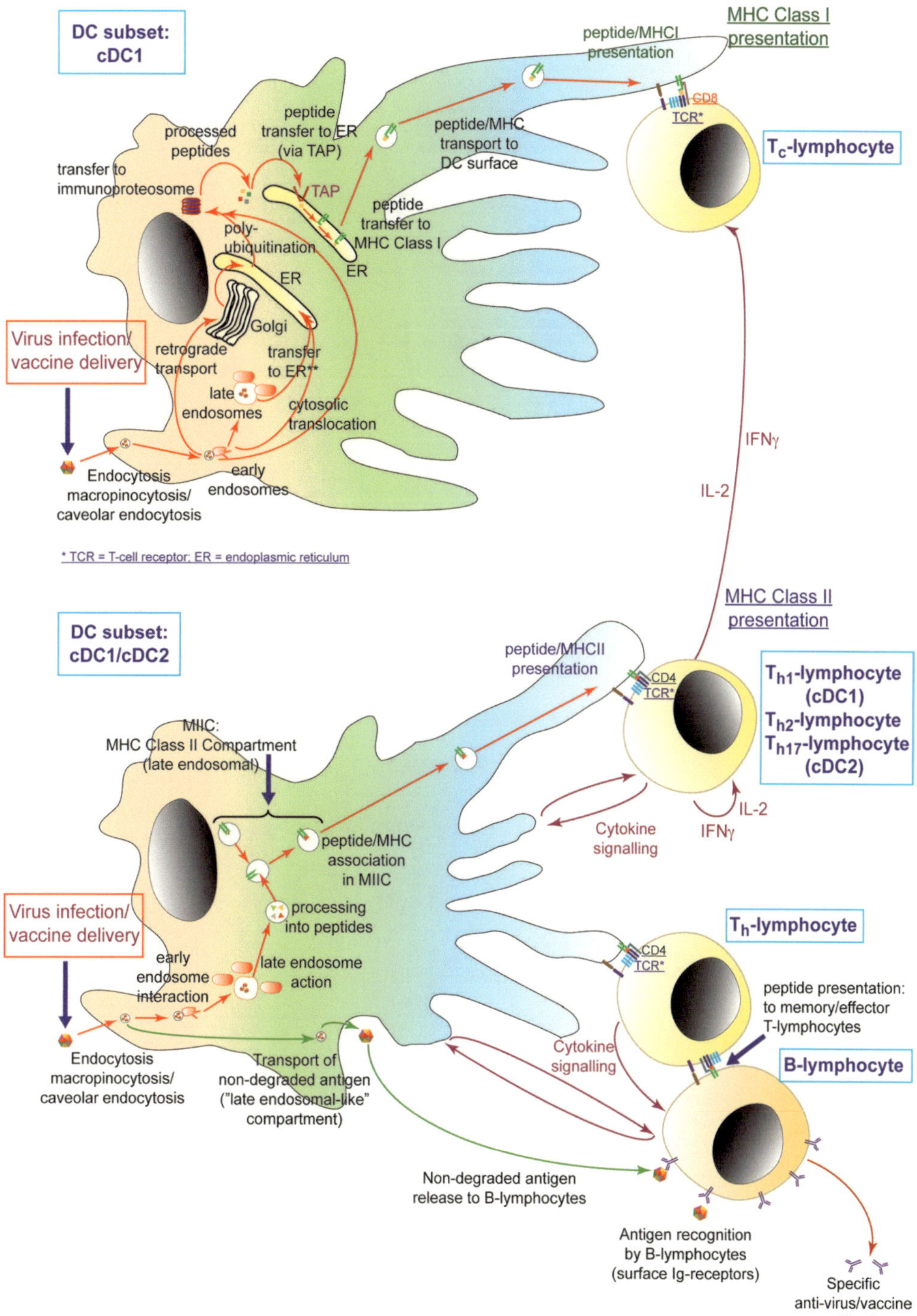

Figure 1. Generalised overview of the two main cDC subsets—cDC1 and cDC2—following endocytosis of virus or vaccine; processing pathways of endocytosed material leading into MHC Class I and MHC Class II presentation of the antigenic peptides to T-lymphocytes; delivery of antigen to B-lymphocytes; resultant initiation of antigen-specific immune defences and antibody production.

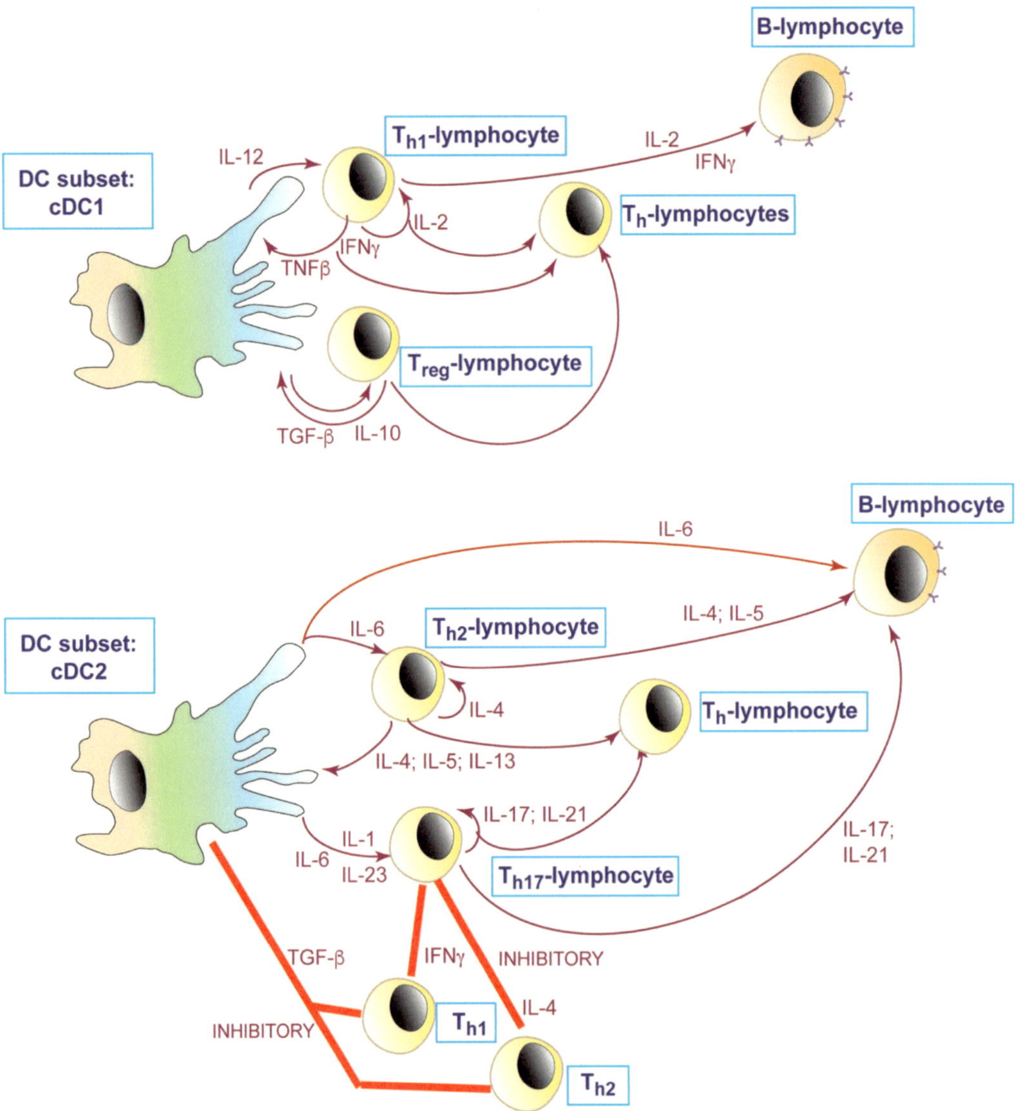

Figure 2. DC subset interaction with different T-lymphocyte subsets. Following processing and presentation of the derived antigen peptides to antigen-specific T_h- or T_{reg}-lymphocytes, the patterns of cytokine communications are shown. These are important for defining the characteristics of the developing immune response. The endocytic processes involved are likely to be clathrin-independent endocytosis such as macropinocytosis, caveolar endocytosis or phagocytosis.

transport though the Golgi complex into the endoplasmic reticulum (ER) (**Figure 1**; **Figure 3** pathway (c)) [9, 26–29].

Further insight into the versatility of DC endocytic process has come from studies on initiation of RNA virus replication [25]. These have identified certain points of convergence with cross-presentation of protein-based vaccines, and thus initiation of RNA vaccine translation of encoded antigens [9]. Importantly, both cross-presentation of antigen and initiation of endocytosed

http://dx.doi.org/10.5772/67779

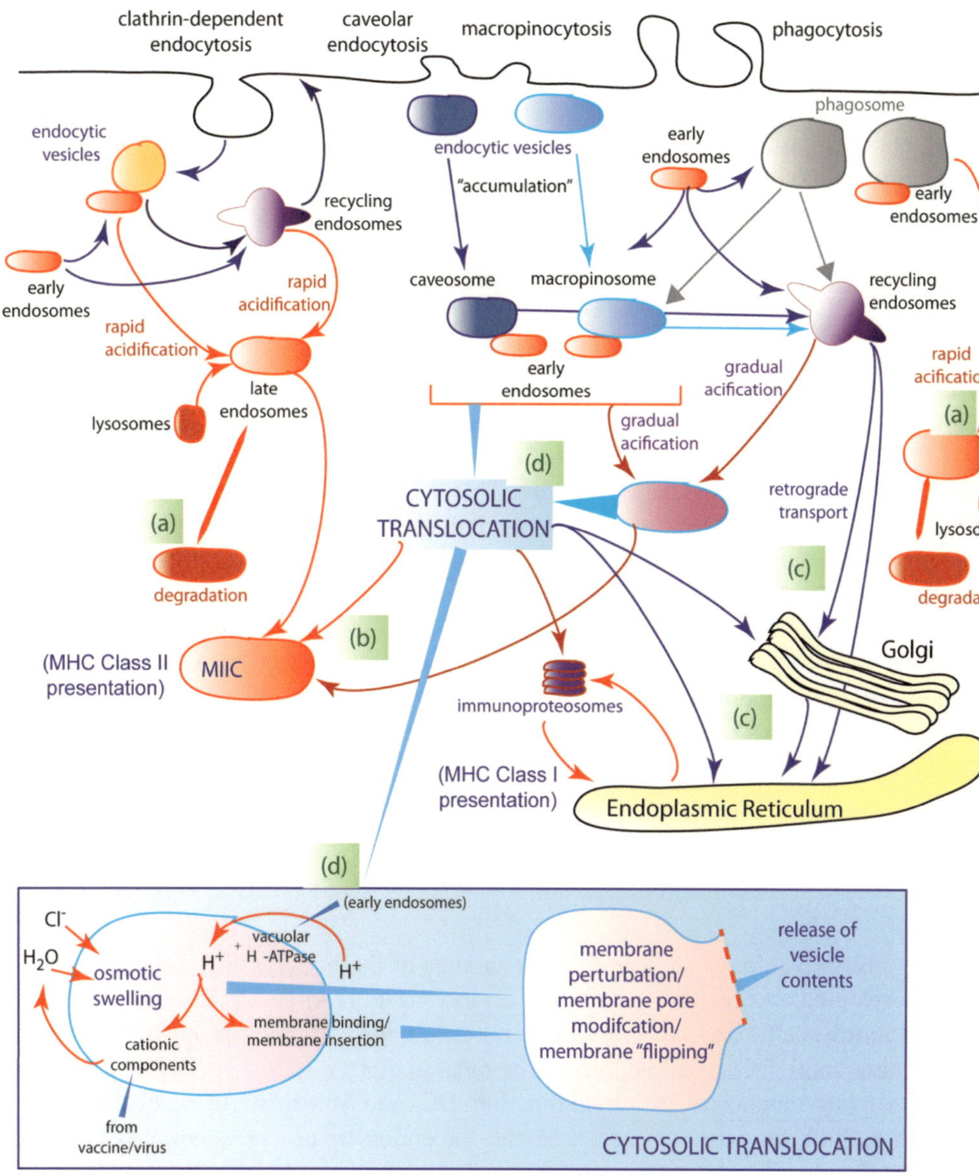

Figure 3. A schematic representation of the main endocytic processes functional within DCs in terms of processing internalised material for (a) degradation, (b) MHC Class II presentation, (c) MHC Class I presentation and (d) cytosolic release for cross-presentation via the immunoproteasome or translation of RepRNA vaccines. The lower portion of the image highlights certain aspects of endosomal release from endocytic vesicles during the early stages after acidification by interaction with early endosomes.

RNA translation require DC endocytosis leading into cytosolic translocation. Endocytosis for cross-presentation delivers exogenous antigen via cytosolic translocation into pathways of polyubiquitination; this directs processing by the immunoproteosome (cross-presentation) for presentation via major histocompatibility complex (MHC) Class I (**Figure 1**, **Figure 3** pathways

(c) and (d)) [9, 30–32]. Similarly, endocytosed vaccine RNA would be delivered by cytosolic translocation into the ribosomal translation sites within the cell for translation of the encoded vaccine antigens [9, 25].

Cationic entities, particularly in a vaccine formulation, have been characterized for their capacity to promote endocytic vesicle perturbation towards cytosolic translocation [9, 13]. Yet, there are other considerations. Initiation of a virus infectious process may involve the viral membrane (with enveloped viruses) or virus surface proteins; thus, cytosolic translocation can be facilitated by membrane fusion and 'flipping', or through formation of ion channels and elaborating membrane pores for delivery of the RNA genome [25]. Application of this knowledge has recently been employed with synthetic biodegradable nanoparticulate vehicles for enhancing delivery of self-amplifying/replicating RepRNA vaccines to DCs [9, 13, 17–20, 33–35] (**Figure 3** pathway (d)). Whilst success with this approach has been forthcoming with mRNA vaccine delivery to DCs [9, 36, 37], delivery of the larger replicon RepRNA molecules has required additional considerations. This may be due to the likely increased compaction of these larger RNA molecules by the delivery vehicle, but other events important to the virus genome from which RepRNA is derived must be considered, including the role of cellular micro-RNAs (miRNA) and divalent cations. Nonetheless, nanoparticulate delivery technology has been adapted to deliver RepRNA to DCs (see below), leading to promotion of the replicon-encoded antigen translation *in vitro* and *in vivo* [13, 17–20, 33, 34]. The work identified important relationships between the DC endocytic pathways and ultimate induction of immune responses by the nanoparticle-delivered RepRNA, relating to characteristics observed following virus infection.

2. Dendritic cells: sentinels of immune defence

Dendritic cell (DC) subsets are found in many sites of the body, which determines their roles in developing and regulating immune defences (**Figure 4**) [1–12]. Together with MΦ, tissue and mucosal DCs are in the front line for encounter with and response to a virus or vaccine. These 'local' DCs and MΦ initiate the inflammatory response recruiting additional DCs together with monocytes, differentiating into DCs and MΦ, to augment local cell activity (**Figure 4**). Both the receptor repertoire and the endocytic processes employed by DCs and MΦ are closely related. Nonetheless, major distinctions exist, notably the recruitment of lysosomal proteases to the acidifying endocytic pathways is observed earlier and at higher levels in MΦ compared with DCs [38].

Dendritic cells are the central players for effective convalescent immunity, efficacious vaccination and maintenance of tolerance (**Figure 2**; **Figure 4**) [1, 3, 4, 6–8]. They are capable of both MHC Class II presentation (**Figure 1**; **Figure 2**), MHC Class I presentation, cross-presentation (**Figure 1**) [30, 32, 39–43] and antigen delivery to B lymphocytes (**Figure 1**) [44, 45], as well as regulating immune responsiveness and immune tolerance (**Figure 2**; **Figure 4**) [6, 46–53]. Therein lie two important aspects of DC biology—their high capacity for endocytosis together with the diverse network of routes employed (**Figure 3**) and different subsets tend

http://dx.doi.org/10.5772/67779

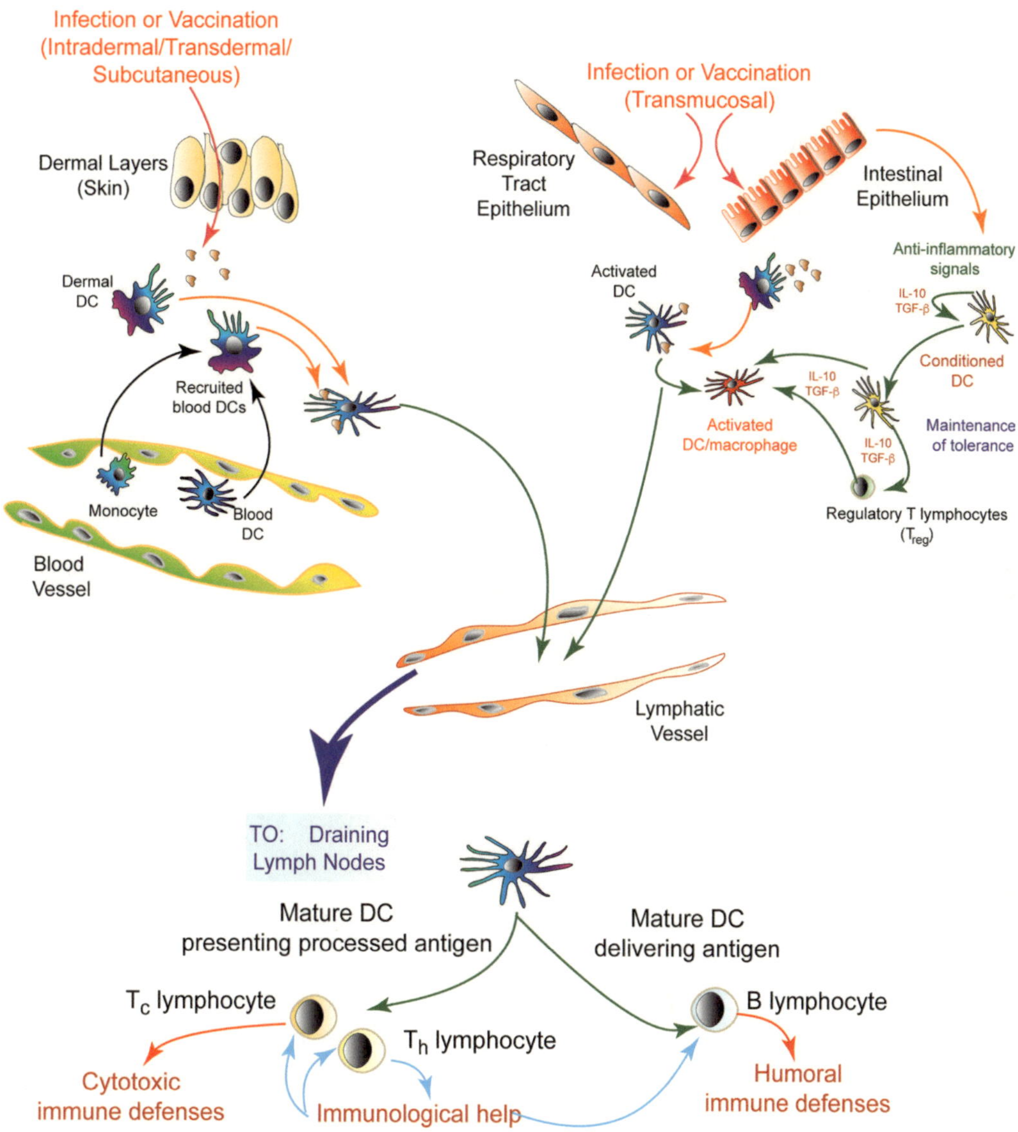

Figure 4. Dendritic cell subsets can be defined with respect to their sites of 'residence' in the body, wherein they act as sentinels for sampling the environment, to maintain tolerance and respond to 'foreign' material posing a 'danger' to the host. This is particularly notable at mucosal surfaces for controlling local tolerance through anti-inflammatory processes, while ensuring responsiveness against pathogenic entities and mucosal vaccines.

to dominate particular processes [3–5, 9, 12, 21–23, 54–56]. Although particular endocytic routes may dominate under certain interactions between DCs and virus or vaccine, more than one endocytic route will often be involved [9, 22, 56]. Indeed, using SVLP vaccines [14, 15], multiple endocytic routes have been identified. While macropinocytosis played a major role, additional endocytic routes were operative, as observed with mature DCs no longer employing macropinocytic activity [14].

3. Application of multiple endocytic pathways

Combining studies on both virus infection of and vaccine delivery to DCs have led to the creation of new vaccine formulations, such as SVLP vaccines [14, 15] and the self-amplifying RepRNA vaccines [9, 17–19, 33]. While clathrin-mediated endocytosis has often been implicated with both virus infection and vaccine delivery [9, 22, 25, 55–57], the rapidity of the process and levels of enzymatic activity therein would favour a more degradative pathway, rather than one promoting antigen processing or RNA-release for translation. Certainly, rapid clathrin-mediated endocytosis would create a detrimental environment to the survival of both RNA viruses and RNA vaccines (**Figure 3**, pathway (a)).

Accordingly, antigen must be processed to reach either the MHC Class I or MHC Class II assembly sites for appropriate antigen presentation (**Figure 3**, pathways (b), to (d)); RNA must be processed to reach the ribosomal translation machinery. Both exogenous antigen and RNA must avoid the degradative capacities of the late endosomes and, in particular, the lysosomes. Antigen being processed through the maturing endosomal system has to target the MHC Class II compartment (MIIC), for MHC Class II presentation, providing processing rather than degradation by lysosomes. With MHC Class I presentation, endocytosed exogenous antigen has to transfer from the endocytic pathway to the cytosol—cytosolic translocation. This facilitates the cross-presentation processing pathway via immunoproteasomes. An important characteristic is that the cytosolic translocation must be effected at a relatively early stage of endosome-mediated acidification of endocytic vesicles (see below). As for RNA, from viruses or vaccines, the cytosolic transfer for translation has to occur before the maturing endosomal system becomes too degradative; that is viral RNA genomes and RNA vaccines must escape the maturing endosomal system while still capable of translating [9, 38, 40, 43, 58].

While these differential processing pathways of DCs are important for ensuring efficient provision of antigen in the correct form for immune defence development, an additional process is essential, namely, endocytosis leading into 'danger' signalling. From within the endosomal system, this involves toll-like receptor (TLR)-containing endosome-like structures, which in turn are unlikely to provide antigen presentation and certainly detrimental to RNA release for translation. Following cytosolic translocation of RNA, danger signalling can be effected through cytosolic detectors such as the retinoic acid-inducible gene-I (RIG-I) family of helicases (see below). Accordingly, DCs employ different endocytic mechanisms and pathways to ensure correct processing of antigen, appropriate cytosolic translocation for cross-presentation, cytosolic translocation of RNA for translation, and appropriate delivery of antigen-based or RNA-based entities to the 'danger' signalling pathways.

4. Dendritic cell sensing

With DCs being an important sentinel of the immune system, the receptors on these cells play critical roles in different aspects of host environment surveillance (**Figure 5**). On the one side,

http://dx.doi.org/10.5772/67779

particular DC receptors are more involved in pathogen or vaccine uptake. In addition to this, DC handling of material 'foreign' to the host can lead to 'danger' recognition, which effectively determines immune activation as opposed to tolerance induction. Dendritic cell pattern recognition receptors (PRRs) recognise pathogen-associated or danger-associated molecular patterns (PAMPs and DAMPs), playing major roles in this recognition and ultimate signalling of the DCs.

Dendritic cell receptor ligation determines the manner by which DCs endocytose and the outcome of the DC activity. One important consequence of ligating certain receptors is the induction of inflammatory reactions (see **Figure 2** and **Figure 4**), the characteristics of which relate to the receptors involved [5, 59, 60]. While PRRs such as toll-like receptors (TLRs), complement receptors and mannose-binding receptors (**Figure 5**) are important for inflammatory responses, both these and other receptors including other C-type lectins, integrins and CD44 can enhance 'foreign' material binding to and internalisation by the cells into endocytic processing pathways [5, 9, 61–63]. For example, ligation of TLRs, siglecs, galectins and CD14 can promote antigen uptake as well as activating innate defence processes, either alone or in co-operation with C-type lectins or integrins [9, 64, 65]. Moreover, different DC receptors can promote uptake into different endocytic pathways. For example, cholera toxin may be targeted to caveolar endocytic pathways and the ER, whereas autocrine mobility factor associates more with the ER [66]. While simian virus 40 (SV40) also targets to the ER, both this and cholera toxin are observed in recycling endosomes prior to retrograde transport into the Golgi and ER [26–29].

In addition to DC sensing their environment via cell surface PRRs such as TLR2 heterodimers and TLR4, endocytosed material can also be sensed. Vesicular TLR2 can detect lipopeptides

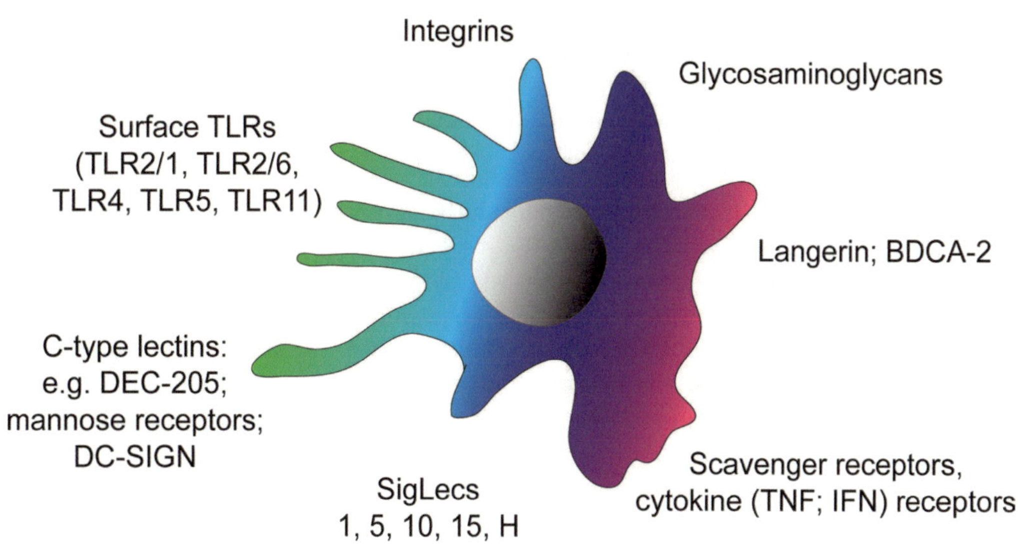

Figure 5. Examples of known DC receptors, demonstrating their wide range of capacities for sampling the host environment. These receptors also offer the potential for targeting vaccines to DC, particularly with the new synthetic vaccines employing nanoparticulate delivery vehicles.

buried deep within bacterial cell walls following endosomal degradation of the latter to expose the lipopeptides. This was proven using SVLPs carrying TLR2 ligands within their hydrophobic cores [15]. By employing such SVLPs, there was no influence of interaction with cell surface TLR2 heterodimers, as is the case with bacteria and yeast particles through the lipoteichoic acid and peptidoglycan moieties in their cell walls.

Additional intracellular PRRs are also involved in detecting 'foreign' RNA—vesicular TLR3 and TLR7, and cytosolic sensors including helicases [67–69]. RNA sensing is an important issue for RNA virus infection and RNA vaccine delivery. Pathogen-associated molecular patterns (PAMPs) associated with 'foreign' RNA are generally formed through RNA modifications or secondary structures not normally found within the cells. TLR3 and TLR7 can respond to dsRNA and ssRNA structures on the 'foreign' RNA, respectively, such PRR activity being linked with processing via the endosomal system. Yet the RNA associated with RNA virus infections as well as with delivery of RNA vaccine can be translocated to the cytosol through action of the virus or vaccine particles (see below). Under these conditions, cytosolic sensors become important for detecting RNA-associated PAMPs.

5. Cytosolic PRR activity

Cytosolic helicases can detect RNA translocated to the cytosol from vesicular structures. The cytosolic helicases of the RIG-I-like receptors (RLRs) family recognise RNA-associated PAMPs through their helicase domain and C-terminal repressor domain (RD); the consequential triggering of intracellular signalling cascades is effected via the caspase-recruitment (CARD) domains [70]. As with the RNA-sensing TLRs, RLRs can recognise PAMPs associated with either ssRNA or dsRNA. The latter come from the dsRNA intermediates derived from replicating viral genomic RNA or RepRNA; single-stranded RNA molecules can also form double-stranded sequences during the hairpin-folding for their secondary structures, the length of which will determine their detection as PAMPs [71]. In addition to such structures, RNA bearing a 5′-triphosphate will also be sensed by helicases.

Within the RLR family, RIG-I responds to both short dsRNA sequences and ssRNA bearing a 5′-triphosphate; MDA-5 responds more to long dsRNA [70]. 5′-triphosphate structures are often required by positive-strand RNA viruses (termed 'positive strand' due to the capacity of the viral genome to function as an mRNA) to ensure ribosomal entry for translation. During the replication of RNA viruses and RepRNA, dsRNA 'replicative intermediates' are formed to generate progeny ssRNA (hence the 'self-amplifying term associated with RepRNA vaccines). Thus, DCs endocytosing RNA viruses or vaccines capable of self-amplification would respond to dsRNA replicative intermediates, in addition to the double stranded secondary structures in the endocytosed RNA, and 5′-triphosphate if present.

This 'danger' sensing of RNA structures provides a good example of the divergence displayed by different DC subsets, and the influence on the cytokine profiles induced. Plasmacytoid DCs (pDCs) tend more to use TLR3 and TLR7 sensing; other cells will employ the cytosolic sensors of RLRs and oligomerization domain (NOD)-like receptors (NLRs), which also respond to dsRNA structures [70]. While RLR- and TLR-mediated activation leads to type I interferon and pro-inflammatory cytokine production, dependent on the DC type, NLR-mediated activation favours IL-1β induction; it is also important to note that dsRNA sensing by NLRs is involved in the regulation of the induced responses [70].

Thus, 'danger' recognition can lead to particular cytokine profiles dependent on the sensing receptor and DC subset involved. The pDC sensing of RNA by TLR3 and TLR7 (and DNA by TLR8/9) leads to the production of notably high levels of IFN-α and TNF, particularly in response to infection. In addition to their anti-viral properties, these cytokines provide the necessary signals to promote appropriate cDC maturation, essential for ensuring that antigen presentation to lymphocytes promotes the development of an antigen-specific adaptive immune response. However, induction of cytokine production by DCs, cDCs and pDCs, will not always prove beneficial in promoting effective immune defence. For example, viruses such as influenza virus and haemorrhagic disease viruses can induce excessive levels of IFN-α and other inflammatory cytokines, leading to the so-called cytokine storm and subsequent immunopathological problems [72–75]. Even viruses not renowned for inducing such events can be prove troublesome. For example, foot-and mouth disease virus infection in pigs can increase IL-10 production by DCs, with a consequential negative influence on antigen presentation and T-lymphocyte activation; in contrast, immune complexes with foot and mouth disease virus are potent inducers of IFN-α by pDCs [76, 77].

Such studies on virus infection of DCs have helped to define conditions beneficial for the host, and therefore what is required for efficacious vaccination. Dendritic cell cytokine induction is certainly critical for inducing maturation of cDCs, an essential requirement for both migration into lymph nodes and efficient presentation of antigen leading to activation of T-lymphocyte responses [2, 7, 10, 62]. Overall, one should consider that targeting slower endocytic processing pathways rather than targeting the more rapid and degradative pathways would prove crucial.

6. Comparative endocytic processes within DCs

The aforementioned differences between MΦ and DCs give an important insight into the characteristics of endocytic processing. Dendritic cells degrade endocytosed material at slower rates, with an overall less acidic phagosomal/endosomal pH than MΦ [38]. These characteristics relate to the different biological roles of the two cell types. On the one hand, DCs are more important for processing and delivering antigen to activate lymphocyte responses. Conversely, MΦ play a more significant role in innate immune cell defence, notably pertinent in the removal and destruction of infectious pathogens, as well as entities presenting a danger to the host, such as damaged or dying cells. Nonetheless, these roles are neither absolute nor mutually exclusive; DCs and MΦ interact during inflammatory responses and the recruitment of cells, including additional DCs, MΦ, T-lymphocytes and NK cells.

The slower endocytic processes noted with DCs would certainly be favourable for efficient antigen processing leading to presentation, as well as cytosolic translocation for cross-presentation or facilitating RNA translation (see **Figure 3**). Yet, despite the difference in the cellular components and the rate of endocytic processing, both clathrin-dependent and clathrin-independent pathways show a major relationship. Although some employ dynamin while other pathways are dynamin-independent [21–23, 78–80], both processing pathways can lead to interaction with early endosomes (**Figure 3**). This provides acidification by vacuolar H^+-ATPase activity and enzyme-mediated degradation within the endocytic vesicle. The important difference between the rapid clathrin-dependent endocytosis and slower clathrin-independent routes is the rate at which endosomal interaction and acidification occur [21–23, 55–57]. The clathrin-independent endocytic processes, such as macropinocytosis, lipid raft-dependent and caveolae-mediated endocytosis, are notably active with DCs, facilitating processing of antigen for presentation via MHC Class II [9, 23, 54, 56, 57]. Moreover, slower processes support retention of endocytosed material at the earlier stages of endosomal maturation in DCs for longer periods, increasing the potential for cytosolic translocation. Nonetheless, clathrin-dependent endocytic processes have been employed by viruses to promote initiation of their infectious cycle. Ebola virus, coronaviruses and certain mammalian reoviruses employ clathrin-dependent endocytosis for their infections [81]. Other viruses, such as influenza virus, employ both clathrin-dependent [82] and clathrin-independent pathways, the latter proving also caveolin-independent. Certain bacterial toxins are also endocytosed by clathrin-dependent and clathrin-independent pathways [26–28, 83–85].

6.1. Macropinocytosis in dendritic cells

The clathrin-independent macropinocytosis relates to clathrin-dependent endocytosis in concentrating receptors upon internalisation, although macropinosomes are more heterogeneous in size—up to 5 μm diameter. The function of macropinocytosis also impacts strongly on DCs in their role of antigen processing for presentation to the adaptive immune system. Both DCs and MΦ employ macropinocytosis more efficiently than other cells [86], through their application of aquaporin channels to sample the environment [87], exhibiting fluid phase uptake up to 40% of their cell volume [88]. Macropinocytic activity is also important with respect to the aforementioned maturation of DCs which is essential for efficient antigen presentation to T-lymphocytes. Aquaporins are down-regulated in mature DCs, relating to the observed reduction in macropinocytosis [87]. In contrast, maturation of DCs does not affect other receptor-mediated endocytosis processes.

The fate of macropinosomes is also particular to DCs and MΦ, wherein macropinosomes fuse with early endosomes soon after formation (**Figure 3**). Macropinosomes acquire Rab7, exchanging their membrane content with late endosomes as they are transported to a more perinuclear area [89]. This contrasts with non-immune cells, such as epithelial and fibroblastic cells, wherein macropinosomes tend to remain more isolated from endosomes and lysosomes, fusing back with the plasma membrane to release their content into the extracellular space [90, 91].

Clearly, macropinocytosis is an important component for facilitating antigen capture by DCs and MΦ. In the context of antigen processing and presentation, the macropinocytosed antigens are observed in endocytic vesicles and macropinosome-like structures rich in MHC Class II molecules (**Figure 3**, pathway (b)) [88, 92]. Antigens endocytosed via macropinocytosis can also be presented on MHC Class I molecules—the cross-presentation pathway following antigen translocation to the cytosol for processing via the immunoproteosome (**Figure 3**, pathway (c)) [93]. Yet, DCs employ other endocytic pathways in addition to macropinocytosis (**Figure 3**). Caveolin-dependent endocytosis is important, as is lipid raft-mediated endocytosis, although the latter can be associated with both macropinocytosis and caveolar endocytosis. Clathrin-independent endocytosis routes in the absence of caveolin may become solely dependent on lipid rafts for intracellular trafficking.

6.2. Processing macropinosomes and other endocytic processes

Following the endocytosis, early endosomes associating with endocytic vesicles are considered key players for cargo sorting (see **Figure 3**). An important bifurcation of endocytic pathways occurs at this stage, channelling into Rab11$^+$ recycling endosomes or into intra-luminal vesicles of multi-vesicular endosomes (MVEs; or MVBs for multi-vesicular bodies). Via these latter structures, processing will ultimately lead into late endosomes and lysosomes. Many late endosomes are involved in the degradative pathway resulting in association of lysosomes and degradation of the cargo, but a late endosome-related structure is essential for MHC Class II presentation—the MHC Class II compartment (MIIC). Late endosomes may also be associated with transfer into vesicular structures carrying the internal TLRs. Moreover, the channelling of endocytosed antigen in a relatively intact form for delivery to B-lymphocytes employs late endosome-like structures [44, 45]. Not only macropinocytosis, but also caveolin-dependent endocytosis crosstalk with classical endosomal components [94], including fusion with Rab11$^+$ recycling endosomes—caveolin$^+$ caveosomes are also seen to be sorted from endosomal compartments [95].

Caveolar endocytosis has been noted with particular entities interacting with cells, including albumin [96], tetanus toxin [97], cholera toxin [98] and both polyomavirus and SV40 [99]. The uptake of cholera toxin [100] is particularly noteworthy, considering the involvement of the recycling endosomes with caveolar endocytosis. The B subunit of the toxin is responsible for cell entry following binding to the monosialotetrahexosylganglioside (GM1) found in lipid rafts and caveolae. Although the CTB subunit can associate with clathrin-dependent endocytic vesicles and clathrin-coated pits [101], and inhibition of clathrin-mediated endocytosis reduces cholera toxin internalisation [98, 102], the toxin activity it is not dependent on clathrin-dependent endocytosis [102]. For this, the cholera toxin must be delivered into Golgi complex, which requires retrograde transport from the recycling endosomes (**Figure 3**) [26–28]. In fact cholera toxin can be endocytosed by different routes, but is ultimately delivered from recycling endosomes to Golgi complex via a clathrin-independent pathway [100, 103], as is shiga toxin [104]. It is also likely that viruses such as polyomavirus and SV40 may require similar routes of entry [105]. Overall, the important lesson from these studies is the capacity of DCs to employ different endocytic routes, some particular to certain antigenic materials, and others being employed in combination. Whether the DCs employ a particular endocytic pathway or a number of different routes, the outcome is dependent on the pathway employed and therefore influences how the DCs handle the endocytosed cargo.

7. Cytosolic translocation in dendritic cells

As mentioned above, retrograde transport from recycling endosomes into the Golgi and ER (see **Figure 3**) is an important pathway for the B subunit of cholera and shiga toxins to promote cytosolic translocation of the A subunit [26–28]. Polyomavirus and SV40 also translocate from the ER for initiation of their replicative cycle [105]. These pathways can be employed by DCs for the cytosolic translocation leading to cross-presentation of exogenous antigen.

Following the retrograde pathway, cytosolic translocation is likely dependent on protein-protein interactions facilitating entry into the cytosol, as observed with the mechanisms employed by cholera and shiga toxins and members of the polyomaviridae. Association of ER membranes with endocytic vesicles can insert the ER dislocon, leading to antigen associated with ER-like structures and subsequent entry into cross-presentation pathways [39, 43].

Yet, DCs can also employ non-retrograde pathways–relatively slow clathrin-dependent endocytosis or the clathrin-independent macropinocytosis–for cytosolic translocation leading into the cross-presentation pathways. This cytosolic translocation displays distinctive characteristics dependent on which of the endocytic routes is employed, but requires interaction with early endosomes. The neutral pH environment of the ER and proteolytic activity therein is clearly distinctive from the events associated with clathrin-dependent and clathrin-independent endocytosis involving endosomal interactions. With the latter, the early endosomes provide membrane vacuolar H^+-ATPases promoting acidification of the endocytic vesicles, an essential event for facilitating cytosolic translocation from these arms of the endocytic processing pathways.

An important influence on the outcome of endocytic vesicles interacting with early endosomes is the role of cationic elements within virus particles or vaccine delivery vehicles. Cationic entities, associated with peptide, lipid or saccharide structures can provide what has been referred to as the 'proton sponge' or 'pH-buffering' effect (**Figure 3**, pathway (d)) [106, 107]. The vacuolar H^+-ATPase activity from early endosomes pumps protons into the endocytic vesicle leading to this proton sponge effect. For example, protonable amines behave as buffering agents by readily accepting protonation [108]. Histidine- and arginine-rich molecules, as well as histidine residues, can also initiate the proton sponge effect through protonation of imidazole rings [106, 107]. By increasing ion and water uptake into the endocytic vesicles, the protonation events increase osmotic pressure leading to vesicular swelling and membrane destabilisation, allowing cytosolic release of the vesicle contents. However, disruption of the endocytic vesicles would prove a relatively destructive process, and are not ideal for the intracellular environment. A more physiologically appropriate process can be seen when analysing histidine- and arginine-rich peptides and polymers, with which cytosolic translocation can be promoted through interaction with the anionic vesicular membrane [107]. This is particularly notable with amphiphilic peptides. Binding at the edge of membrane pores can reduce internal membrane tension, while insertion into the vesicular membrane can reduce chain length to create internal membrane tension [106, 109]. Cationic lipids will also influence cytosolic translocation by ionic paring with phosphatidylserine in endocytic vesicle membrane [110]. This promotes electrostatic interactions and decreases membrane curvature, potentially with conversion from a lamellar to a non-lamellar phase.

Regardless of which endocytosis pathway is employed by the DC to process internalised cargo, the outcome will be either destruction or processing. For the latter, this can lead through the maturing endosomal system for MHC Class II presentation, or can involve one of the pathways of cytosolic translocation for MHC Class I presentation. With RNA viruses and RNA vaccines, the latter pathways would be more favourable, promoting delivery of the RNA to the ribosomal translation machinery. In the case of RNA vaccines, this translation would provide the antigens for direction into the immunoproteosome from the ER, or probably via autophagy into the endosomal system for delivery to the MIIC.

8. Dendritic cell endocytosis leading to MHC Class I or MHC Class II presentation

As mentioned above, MΦ with DCs employ common endocytic processes for ultimately distinctive outcomes [38]. While MΦ rapidly recruit and activate lysosomal proteases, leading to rapid degradation of endocytic cargo, the lower acidic endosomal pH and slower acidifying process within DCs favour slower degradation of internalized cargoes. DCs also generate reactive oxygen species in endocytic compartments through the activated NOX2 subunit of NADPH-oxidase, which in turn consume protons and modulate the pH. This rate of endosomal acidification is important for the consequences of the processing pathway, and therefore both directing into the MIIC and cytosolic translocation. Although acidification of the endosomal structures is a characteristic of the so-called endosomal maturation leading into the more destructive late endosomes and lysosomes, the early stages of the endosomal acidification play particularly essential roles for cytosolic translocation from the endosomal compartment. Therefore, a more 'regulated' (in terms of rate) endosomal acidification would facilitate the processing events leading to MHC Class I and MHC Class II presentation. Importantly however, once the acidification falls below a certain pH, the potential for translocation to the cytosol becomes less likely, and the endosomal structures become 'cross-presentation incompetent' [38]. This situation relates to the concomitant decrease of pH and ER-derived proteins, with increased proteolytic activity.

It is now clear that exogenous antigen can be processed into the MHC Class I pathway via 'cross-presentation' pathways [40, 43, 57, 58, 111] which is important for activating the Tc lymphocytes of cytotoxic CMI (see **Figure 1**). Consideration of these characteristics has also proven valuable for understanding the requirement of endocytosed RNA and RNA viruses for cytosolic translocation (see **Figure 3**, pathway (d)). Moreover, the division of labour associated with different DC subsets is an important consideration when cytosolic translocation is required. Participation of different DC receptors leading to endocytosis is influential, defining the form of endocytosis and relative role played by retrograde transport into the ER [43].

When the receptor and endocytic targeting deliver into early compartments such as recycling endosomes, both MHC Class I and Class II presentation can ensue; delivery into and interaction with later endosomal compartments lead to a domination of MHC Class II presentation [38, 112]. Yet, transport of the endocytosed material down a particular pathway favouring MHC Class I or MHC Class II processing is not absolute. For example, material being transported towards an MHC Class I presentation pathway can be transferred into autophagic vesicles for delivery into the MHC Class II presentation pathway.

Overall, it can be considered that processing antigen for association with MHC Class I molecules is a less acidic process compared with the pathway leading to MHC Class II presentation. A good example of this is the aforementioned relative neutral pH of the retrograde pathway though the ER. Another example is seen with cytosolic translocation from early endosomal structures. The initial lowering of endocytic vesicle pH is important, but as mentioned above this is limited by the 'point of no return' within the acidifying endosomal compartment, beyond which the conditions render translocation less likely [38, 43, 113]. Therefore, cytosolic translocation must arise before the more degradative processes of the late endosomes have taken charge.

As mentioned above, not only antigen, but also viruses employ different endocytic pathways to initiate their replicative cycles. While polyomaviruses and SV40 translocate from the ER for this purpose, numerous other viruses require the acidifying endosomal system to initiate their replication. The endosomes provide pH-dependent modifications of viral surface proteins. By such means, endosomal membrane modulation is promoted leading to cytosolic release of the viral genome; in the case of positive strand RNA viruses, the genome functions as a mRNA by interacting directly with the cellular translation machinery; in the case of negative strand viruses, the viral genome is associated with the nucleocapsid carrying the polymerase, the polymerase generating the 'positive strand' to function as an mRNA. Endosomal membrane modulation can result from fusion between the endosomal and viral membranes, as with influenza virus, or re-arrangement of viral proteins to form ion channels and pores in the endosomal membrane, as with picornaviruses and flaviviruses [25]. Related to the former (endosomal membrane fusion), is the work with fusogenic peptides, leading to vesicular membrane destabilisation as the internal pH decreases below 6.0 [107, 109].

These studies on the processes employed by viruses to promote cytosolic translocation have proven useful in the development of processes for the successful delivery of RNA vaccines. In this context, the delivery of self-amplifying replicon RNA is of particular interest, due to its high potential for vaccine development in the future [9, 13, 17–19, 35, 114]. However, these large RNA molecules have particular requirements, which are more stringent or more obligatory than with smaller RNA molecules such as the oligonucleotides of siRNA and mRNA vaccines.

9. Self-amplifying RNA interaction with dendritic cells

Interest in the development of replicating RNA vaccines has increased during the past two decades, notably in the field of self-amplifying RepRNA technology [9, 13, 18, 114–118]. RepRNA are basically viral genomes lacking at least one gene encoding structural proteins, but retaining the genes encoding the viral polymerase (self-amplification/replication) complex (**Figure 6**), hence termed as 'replicon'. This type of construct permits replication of RNA without the risk of progeny virus production and therefore disease; the vaccine element is

http://dx.doi.org/10.5772/67779

introduced by inserting genes encoding vaccine antigens of interest ('genes of interest' or GOI) into the constructs (**Figure 6**) [9, 13, 18, 20, 114–121]. Development of this technology during the past two decades focussed on packaging the RNA in a virus-like particle or the virus replicon particle (VRP) [9, 115–117]. However, this approach can encounter particular problems such as host immunity against the viral proteins composing the VRP surface structure; production difficulties/expense may also prove an encumbrance due to the requirement for complementing cell lines providing the gene products missing from the replicon so that VRPs will be generated [9]. Replacement of the VRP by biodegradable delivery vehicles would facilitate vaccine production (obviating the need for complementing cells lines), avoid problems of the host immune system neutralising the VRP antigens, and permit more controllable targeting of DCs [9]. This approach was first reported in 2008 (**Figure 7**) [20], with

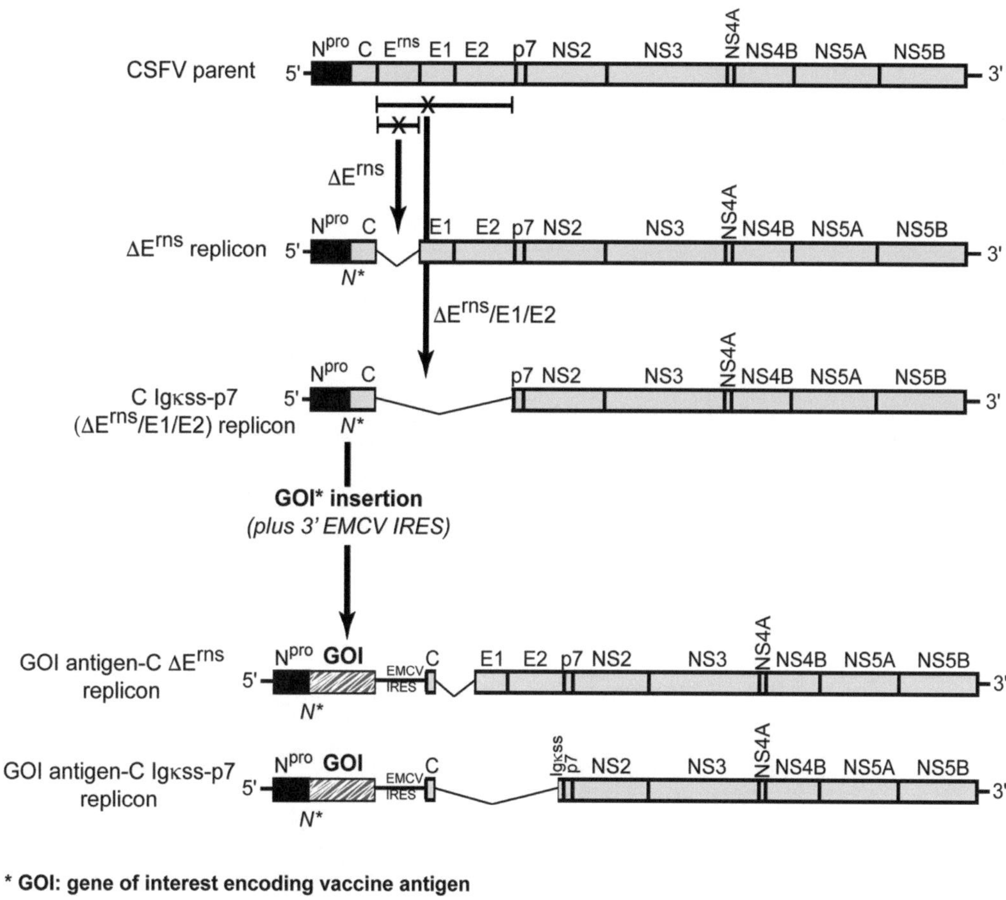

Figure 6. Generation of self-amplifying RepRNA vaccines derived from the CSFV genome, for application with biodegradable nanoparticulate delivery vehicles to target DCs by nanoparticulate vehicles. Two examples are shown: ΔE^{rns} replicon lacking a single (E^{rns}) gene, and C-Igκss-p7 replicon lacking all three structural glycoproteins. NotI endonuclease restriction sites, introduced to facilitate insertion of genes encoding vaccine antigen, are shown at the 3′ end of the N^{pro} leader autoprotease as N*. The site for insertion of the gene of interest (GOI) encoding the vaccine antigen is shown as the hashed box. An additional insertion, an EMCV IRES, is employed to restart the translation which terminates after the GOI.

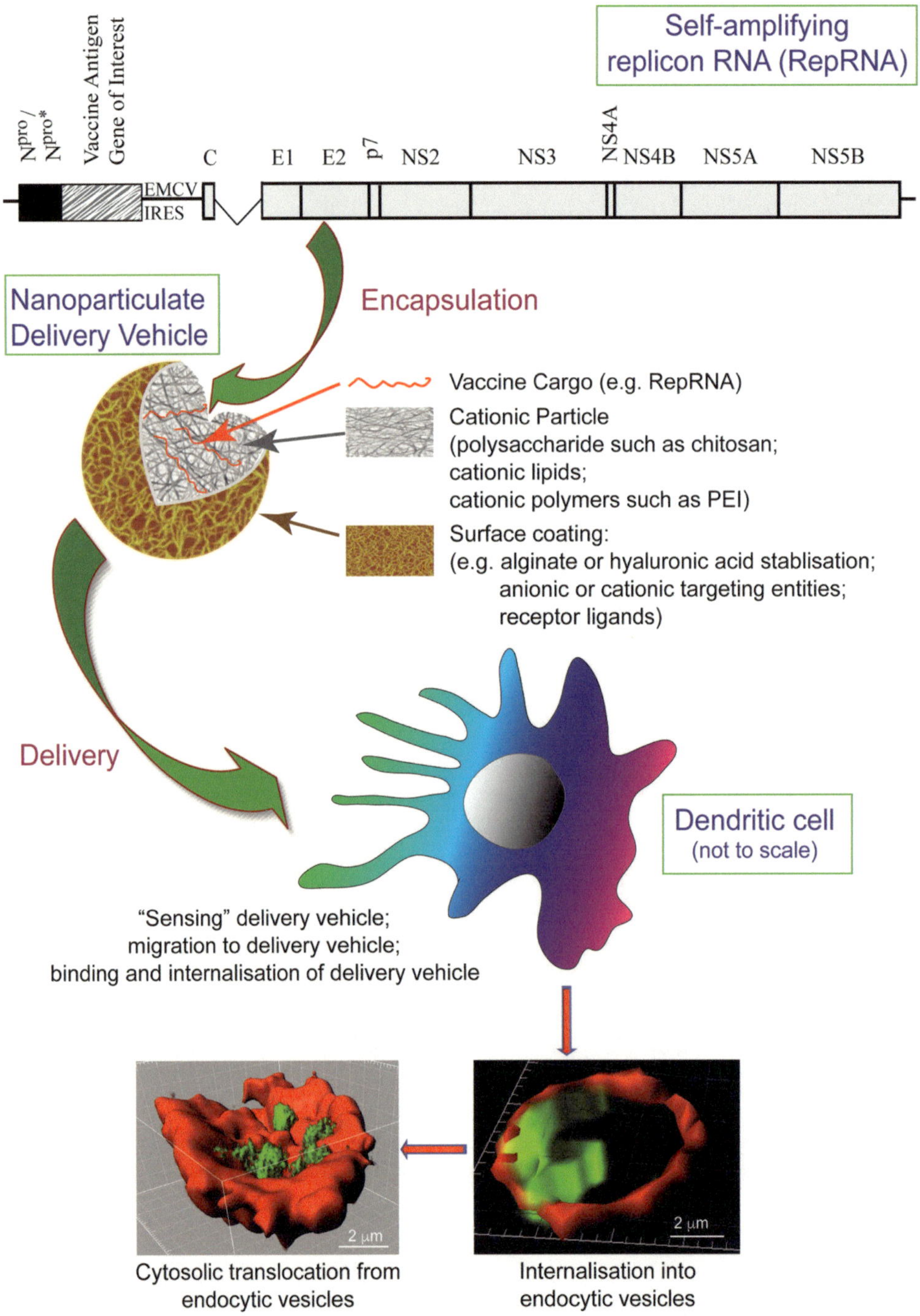

Figure 7. Nanoparticulate delivery of self-amplifying RNA vaccines derived from the CSFV RepRNA. The nanoparticulate delivery vehicle is designed to promote efficient uptake into endocytic vesicles, in which the RepRNA is seen to accumulate. Thereafter, a gradual cytosolic translocation of the RepRNA is observed—essential for RNA delivery to the intracellular site for translation. Thereby, the RepRNA efficiently translates the encoded vaccine antigen of interest, as well as the polymerase complex for replication of the RNA. Insertion of an internal ribosomal entry site (IRES) from EMC virus ensures that translation of the polymerase complex resumes after translation of the vaccine antigen.

increasing evidence of the potential for this methodology forthcoming in more recent years [9, 13, 17–19, 33–35, 114, 122].

RepRNA show the characteristics of the parent virus genome, providing several rounds of replication to increase the number of RNA templates available for translation. By such means, the antigen dosages available for activating humoral immunity and cytotoxic cell-mediated immunity (CMI), as well as the duration of that availability, are enhanced beyond that possible with a more conventional inactivated vaccine approach (**Figure 8**) [9, 13, 17, 18, 20, 114]. Moreover, being replicative in nature enhances their capacity to induce CMI as well as humoral immunity, a characteristic often lacking with inactivated vaccines. Live, attenuated vaccines offer the same advantage due to their replicative nature. A major benefit of RepRNA vaccines is that they do not suffer from the potential risk of reversion to virulence posed by attenuated vaccines, due to their defective nature being unable to produce progeny viruses (**Figure 6**).

Many studies, primarily using VRPs, have employed alphaviruses [115–117]. However, these viruses and the derived RepRNA are cytopathogenic, killing their host cells. The slow processing and retention of antigen typical of DC functionality with respect to inducing robust immune defences would not be favoured by cell death from a cytopathogenic RepRNA, despite their rapid production of antigen. Although delivery of such replicons to epithelial cells would provide antigen indirectly for the DCs, targeting DCs with cytopathogenic replicons is probably not the most effective of approaches. On the other hand, non-cytopathogenic RepRNA vaccines, such as those derived from classical swine fever virus (CSFV) (**Figure 6**) [20, 118], would have higher potential for targeting DCs with the aim of prolonged presence of antigen in these cells (**Figure 7**). While non-cytopathogenic RepRNA should translate antigen slower than cytopathogenic replicons, lower antigen production levels fit well to the DC requirements for prolonged antigen presentation to the adaptive immune system (**Figure 8**).

One major drawback with RepRNA vaccines in general is their high RNase sensitivity. This can be avoided by employing either VRP for delivery or biodegradable nanoparticulate delivery vehicles (**Figure 7**) [9, 13, 18, 20, 114, 123]. From initial efforts in 2003, the concept of RepRNA delivery by biodegradable nanoparticles was developed [20], showing high potential for delivery to DCs (**Figure 7**; **Figure 8**) [9, 13, 18, 114, 17]. Nonetheless, it is now evident that nanoparticulate technology can lead to compaction of RepRNA (**Figure 7**). This was not so apparent with delivery of smaller RNA molecules, such as siRNA and mRNA, only coming to light with the much larger RepRNA molecules. While compaction with the delivery vehicle could interfere with cytosolic translocation, even after the translocation a lack of decompaction would interfere with ribosomal entry and thus translation. Studies turned to the aforementioned importance of protonation within the endocytic vesicle for cytosolic translocation, which could also influence the degree of RNA compaction by the delivery vehicle.

Application of cationic components in the delivery vehicles for RepRNA, such as chitosan cores, cationic lipids and cationic polyplexes (**Figure 7**), has proven successful for enhancing RepRNA delivery [9, 17–19, 33, 35]. Their cationic nature facilitates interaction with RNA and protection from RNases. In addition, they may favour events leading to cytosolic translocation from the endocytic vesicles during the initial phases of early endosome-mediated acidification. Application of additional cationic entities, such as lipids or peptides, may further favour cytosolic delivery and decompaction for translation, potentially by reducing the levels

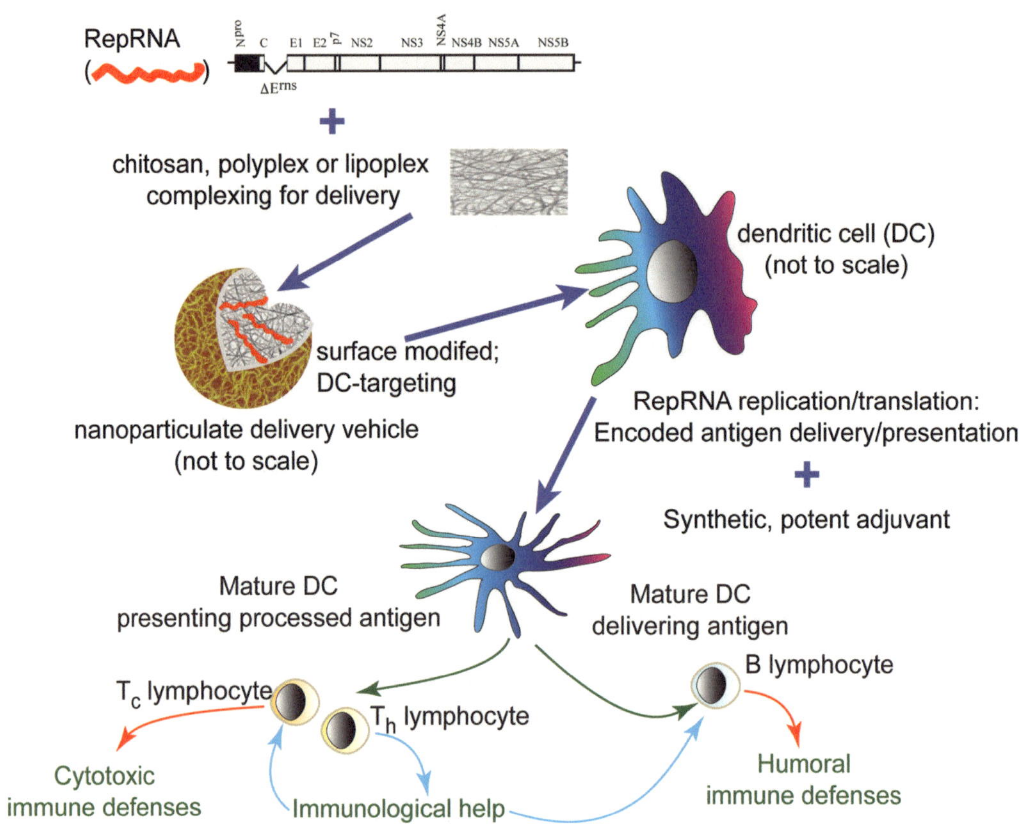

Figure 8. Overview of the procedures for association of RepRNA vaccines with biodegradable nanoparticulate delivery vehicles, targeting DCs to promote induction of both humoral and cytotoxic immune defences.

of compaction obtained by a single cationic entity. Certainly, the presence of cationic lipids in a chitosan-based nanoparticulate delivery vehicle with RepRNA enhanced both the *in vitro* translation of the delivered RNA, and the induction of humoral and CMI immune defences *in vivo* (**Figure 7**; **Figure 8**) [18].

10. Conclusion: dendritic cell endocytosis promoting cross-presentation and RNA translation

Dendritic cells, in particular the cDC1 subset, display the capacity for cross-presentation of exogenous antigenic material (**Figure 1**). Using SVLPs, DCs primarily endocytose these vaccines via macropinocytosis, but an underlying additional endocytic process is also active [14]. While a dominant processing towards MHC Class II presentation is evident, cross-presentation pathways also exist, directing the processing towards MHC Class I presentation [15]. Importantly, these SVLPs do not activate the DC family to promote DC maturation which is essential for efficient induction of adaptive immunity. By modifying the lipopeptide monomers of the SVLPs to carry TLR2 ligands, certain SVLPs are directed into internal TLR2-containing sites for induction of cytokines that are important for DC maturation [15].

The endocytic processes involved in the cytosolic translocation of endocytosed antigen also relate to the delivery of RNA required for translation. RNA vaccines and the genomes of RNA viruses must translocate from the endosomal system or ER (retrograde transport) following endocytosis, to facilitate delivery into cytosolic sites of ribosomal translation (**Figure 3**). With viruses, this can be promoted by the interaction of viral surface proteins with the endosomal membrane, becoming modified upon acidification by early endosome to create ion channels and/or pores in the membrane for cytosolic transfer of the RNA genomes. RNA vaccines can employ similar strategies, when the RNA is packaged within virus-like particles, which can be seen with self-amplifying replicon RNA vaccine delivery as VRPs. With synthetic RNA vaccines, delivered by synthetic nanoparticulate delivery vehicles rather than VRPs or other virus-like particles (**Figure 7**), translocation must occur as the interaction of the RNA with its delivery vehicle becomes weakened to the point of promoting decompaction. There is a critical point of no return, with cytosolic translocation being vital before late endosomal activity dominates. Therefore, the delivery vehicle formulation must facilitate endosomal membrane modification to permit this cytosolic translocation at the appropriate stage of endosomal maturation.

An important issue pertinent to nanoparticle delivery is the size of the delivery vehicle being endocytosed. Size and ionic potential of particles interacting with cells, particularly DCs and MΦ, influence both the endocytic route and how the cell handles internalised material [43, 58]. The smaller the entity the greater the role played by retrograde transport from endocytic vesicles into the ER [58]. Macropinocytosis and caveolar endocytic delivery to the ER may occur without interaction with early endosomes, or shortly after acidification begins (**Figure 3**). Nonetheless, if the delivery vehicle is designed to promote cytosolic translocation and even decompaction when present in an acidifying environment, then RNA delivery should be directed into macropinosomes and caveolar vesicles interacting with early endosomes.

Overall, self-amplifying RepRNA delivery to DCs has high potential for future vaccine development and application, providing controlled and efficacious vaccine delivery, and thus promoting robust immune defence induction (**Figure 8**). Of particular importance is the appropriate application of nanoparticulate delivery vehicle formulations to enhance cytosolic translocation of RNA vaccines in DC, while reducing compaction to ensure ribosomal entry for translation of the encoded vaccine antigens and self-amplification of the replicon RNA.

Acknowledgements

This work was supported by the following: EU FP7 project UniVax [grant number 601738]; Swiss National Science Foundation (SNF) project Replicon-DC [grant number 310030_150008]; Marie-Curie Action FP7-PEOPLE-2009-IAAP, 'Replixcel' [grant number 251420]; EU FP6 project PANFLUVAC [grant number 044115]; ERA-NET projects HCVAX (EuroNanoMed/Swiss

National Science Foundation) [grant number 31NM30-136034/1] and HCRus (University of Geneva, Switzerland) [grant number ERANetRUS 081]; SNF project NANOVACC [grant number 310000_1198828]. We are also most grateful to Brigitte Herrmann for help with the PBMC work and confocal microscopy, and to Andreas Michel and Hans-Peter Lüthi for animal care and bleeding of donor animals for the PBMCs. We are also most grateful to Arin Ghasparian and John A. Robinson (Department of Chemistry, University of Zürich, and Virometix AG, Zurich, Switzerland) for preparing and providing the SVLPs.

Author details

Kenneth C. McCullough[1]* and Rajni Sharma[2]

*Address all correspondence to: kmc.projects1@gmail.com

1 Immunology Department, Institute of Virology and Immunology, Mittelhäusern, Switzerland

2 Immunology-Vaccinology, Faculty of Veterinary Medicine, University of Liège, Liège, Belgium

References

[1] Steinman RM. The dendritic cell system and its role in immunogenicity. Annual Review of Immunology. 1991;**9**:271–296. doi: 10.1146/annurev.iy.09.040191.001415.

[2] Steinman RM, Pack M, Inaba K. Dendritic cells in the T-cell areas of lymphoid organs. Immunological Reviews. 1997;**156**:25–37.

[3] Banchereau J, Steinman RM. Dendritic cells and the control of immunity. Nature. 1998;**392**:245–252. doi: 10.1038/32588.

[4] Banchereau J, Briere F, Caux C, Davoust J, Lebecque S, Liu YJ, Pulendran B, Palucka K. Immunobiology of dendritic cells. Annual Review of Immunology. 2000;**18**:767–811. doi: 10.1146/annurev.immunol.18.1.767.

[5] Medzhitov R, Janeway C, Jr. Innate immune recognition: mechanisms and pathways. Immunological Reviews. 2000;**173**:89–97.

[6] Mellman I, Steinman RM. Dendritic cells: specialized and regulated antigen processing machines. Cell. 2001;**106**:255–258.

[7] Steinman RM, Pope M. Exploiting dendritic cells to improve vaccine efficacy. Journal of Clinical Investigation. 2002;**109**:1519–1526. doi: 10.1172/JCI15962.

[8] Steinman RM, Banchereau J. Taking dendritic cells into medicine. Nature. 2007;**449**:419–426. doi: 10.1038/nature06175.

[9] McCullough KC, Bassi I, Demoulins T, Thomann-Harwood LJ, Ruggli N. Functional RNA delivery targeted to dendritic cells by synthetic nanoparticles. Therapeutic Delivery. 2012;**3**:1077–1099.

[10] Steinman RM, Hemmi H. Dendritic cells: translating innate to adaptive immunity. Current Topics in Microbiology and Immunology. 2006;**311**:17–58.

[11] Geissmann F, Manz MG, Jung S, Sieweke MH, Merad M, Ley K. Development of monocytes, macrophages and dendritic cells. Science. 2010;**327**:656–661.

[12] Steinman RM. Decisions about dendritic cells: past, present, and future. Annual Review of Immunology. 2012;**30**:1–22. doi: 10.1146/annurev-immunol-100311-102839.

[13] McCullough KC, Milona P, Thomann-Harwood L, Demoulins T, Englezou P, Suter R, Ruggli N. Self-amplifying replicon RNA vaccine delivery to dendritic cells by synthetic nanoparticles. Vaccines. 2014;**2**:735–754.

[14] Sharma R, Ghasparian A, Robinson JA, McCullough KC. Synthetic virus-like particles target dendritic cell lipid rafts for rapid endocytosis primarily but not exclusively by macropinocytosis. PLoS One. 2012;**7**:e43248. doi: 10.1371/journal.pone.0043248.

[15] Sharma R, Ghasparian A, Robinson JA, McCullough KC. Dendritic cell sensing of hydrophobic di- and triacylated lipopeptides self-assembled into synthetic virus-like particles. Journal of Immunology. 2017 (under second review).

[16] Ghasparian A, Riedel T, Koomullil J, Moehle K, Gorba C, Svergun DI, Perriman AW, Mann S, Tamborrini M, Pluschke G, Robinson JA. Engineered synthetic virus-like particles and their use in vaccine delivery. Chemical Biochemistry. 2011;**12**:100–109. doi: 10.1002/cbic.201000536.

[17] Demoulins T, Milona P, Englezou PC, Ebensen T, Schulze K, Suter R, Pichon C, Midoux P, Guzman CA, Ruggli N, McCullough KC. Polyethylenimine-based polyplex delivery of self-replicating RNA vaccines. Nanomedicine. 2016;**12**:711–722.

[18] McCullough KC, Bassi I, Milona P, Suter R, Thomann-Harwood L, Englezou P, Démoulins T, Ruggli N. Self-replicating replicon-RNA delivery to dendritic cells by chitosan-nanoparticles for translation In vitro and in vivo. Molecular Therapy Nucleic Acids. 2014;**3**:e173.

[19] McCullough KC, Tirelli N. Next generation vaccines; knocking on cell's door. Pan European Networks: Science and Technology. 2012;**4**:108–109.

[20] Tratschin JD, Ruggli N, McCullough KC. Pestivirus replicons providing an RNA-based viral vector system. PCT/EP2009/003892; WO 2009146867; US 2011/0189224. 2008.

[21] Conner SD, Schmid SL. Regulated portals of entry into the cell. Nature. 2003;**422**:37–44. doi: 10.1038/nature01451.

[22] Kumari S, Mg S, Mayor S. Endocytosis unplugged: multiple ways to enter the cell. Cell Research. 2010;**20**:256–275. doi: 10.1038/cr.2010.19.

[23] Sandvig K, Pust S, Skotland T, van Deurs B. Clathrin-independent endocytosis: mechanisms and function. Current Opinion in Cell Biology. 2011;**23**:413–420. doi: 10.1016/j.ceb.2011.03.007.

[24] Scott CC, Vacca F, Gruenberg J. Endosome maturation, transport and functions. Seminars in Cell and Developmental Biology. 2014;**31**:2–10. doi: 10.1016/j.semcdb.2014.03.034.

[25] Vazquez-Calvo A, Saiz JC, McCullough KC, Sobrino F, Martin-Acebes MA. Acid-dependent viral entry. Virus Research. 2012;**167**:125–137. doi: 10.1016/j.virusres.2012.05.024.

[26] Lu L, Hong W. From endosomes to the trans-Golgi network. Seminars in Cell and Developmental Biology. 2014;**31**:30–39. doi: 10.1016/j.semcdb.2014.04.024.

[27] Mallard F, Antony C, Tenza D, Salamero J, Goud B, Johannes L. Direct pathway from early/recycling endosomes to the Golgi apparatus revealed through the study of shiga toxin B-fragment transport. Journal of Cell Biology. 1998;**143**:973–990.

[28] Sandvig K, van Deurs B. Delivery into cells: lessons learned from plant and bacterial toxins. Gene Therapy. 2005;**12**:865–872. doi: 10.1038/sj.gt.3302525.

[29] Soldati T, Schliwa M. Powering membrane traffic in endocytosis and recycling. Nature Reviews Molecular Cell Biology. 2006;**7**:897–908. doi: 10.1038/nrm2060.

[30] Schuette V, Burgdorf S. The ins-and-outs of endosomal antigens for cross-presentation. Current Opinion in Immunology. 2014;**26**:63–68. doi: 10.1016/j.coi.2013.11.001.

[31] Shete HK, Prabhu RH, Patravale VB. Endosomal escape: a bottleneck in intracellular delivery. The Journal of Nanoscience and Nanotechnology. 2014;**14**:460–474.

[32] Zehner M, Burgdorf S. Regulation of antigen transport into the cytosol for cross-presentation by ubiquitination of the mannose receptor. Molecular Immunology. 2013;**55**:146–148. doi: 10.1016/j.molimm.2012.10.010.

[33] Englezou PC, Milona P, Démoulins T, Sapet C, Ebensen T, Guzman C-A, Suter R, Zelphati O, Ruggli N, McCullough K. Cationic lipids efficiently deliver self-amplifying RepRNA for translation in DC and monocytes. Molecular Therapy. 2017; submitted for publication.

[34] McCullough KC, Ruggli N. Inducing Immunity. International Innovation. 2013;**June** 2013:90–92.

[35] Démoulins T, Englezou PC, Milona P, Ruggli N, Tirelli N, Pichon C, Sapet C, Ebensen T, Guzman C-A, McCullough KC. Self-replicating RNA vaccine delivery to dendritic cells. In T. Kramps and K. Elbers (editors). RNA Vaccines: Methods and Protocols. Springer Science+Business Media, New York, 2017; vol 1499; pp 37–75.

[36] Perche F, Benvegnu T, Berchel M, Lebegue L, Pichon C, Jaffrès P-A, Midoux P. Enhancement of dendritic cells transfection in vivo and of vaccintion against B16F10 melanoma with mannosylated histidylated lipopolyplexes loaded with tumor antigen messenger RNA. Nanomedicine. 2011;**7**:445–453.

[37] Pichon C, Midoux P. Mannosylated and histidylated LPR technology for vaccination with tumor antigen mRNA. Methods in Molecular Biology. 2013;**969**:247–274. doi: 10.1007/978-1-62703-260-5_16.

[38] Amigorena S, Savina A. Intracellular mechanisms of antigen cross presentation in dendritic cells. Current Opinion in Immunology. 2010;**22**:109–117.

[39] Ackerman AL, Kyritsis C, Tampé R, Cresswell P. Access of soluble antigens to the endoplasmic reticulum can explain cross-presentation by dendritic cells. Nature Immunology. 2004;**6**:107–113.

[40] Heath W, Belz G, Behrens GMN, Smith CM, Forehan SP, Parish IA, Davey GM, Wilson NS, Carbone FR, Villadangos JA. Cross-presentation, dendritic cell subsets, and the generation of immunity to cellular antigens. Immunological Reviews. 2004;**199**:9–26.

[41] Ikeuchi N, Futami j, Hosoi A, Noji S, Kurachi M, Ueha S, Fujii S-i, Yamada H, Matsushima K, Moriyasu F, Kakimi K. Efficient cross-presentationof soluble exogenous antigens introduced into dendritic cells using a weak-based amphiphilic peptide. Biochemical and Biophysical Research Communications. 2010;**392**(2):217–22 submitted.

[42] Mant A, Chinnery F, Elliott T, Williams AP. The pathway of cross-presentation is influenced by the particle size of phagocytosed antigen. Immunology. 2012;**136**:163–175. doi: 10.1111/j.1365-2567.2012.03558.x.

[43] Monu N, Trombetta ES. Cross-talk between the endocytic pathway and the endoplasmic reticulum in cross-presentationby MHC class I molecules. Current Opinion in Immunology. 2007;**19**:66–72.

[44] Le Roux D, Le Bon A, Dumas A, Taleb K, Sachse M, Sikora R, Julithe M, Benmerah A, Bismuth G, Niedergang F. Antigen stored in dendritic cells after macropinocytosis is released unprocessed from late endosomes to target B cells. Blood. 2011;**119**:95–105.

[45] Wykes M, Pombo A, Jenkins C, MacPherson GG. Dendritic cells interact directly with naive B lymphocytes to transfer antigen and initiate class switching in a primary T-dependent response. Journal of Immunology. 1998;**161**:1313–1319.

[46] Blankenstein T, Schuler T. Cross-priming versus cross-tolerance: are two signals enough? Trends in Immunology. 2002;**23**:171–173.

[47] Duan W, Croft M. Control of regulatory T cells and airway tolerance by lung macrophages and dendritic cells. Annals of the American Thoracic Society. 2014;**11 Suppl 5**:S306-313. doi: 10.1513/AnnalsATS.201401-028AW.

[48] Lewis KL, Reizis B. Dendritic cells: arbiters of immunity and immunological tolerance. Cold Spring Harbor Perspectives in Biology. 2012;**4**:a007401. doi: 10.1101/cshperspect.a007401.

[49] Lutz MB, Kurts C. Induction of peripheral CD4+ T-cell tolerance and CD8+ T-cell cross-tolerance by dendritic cells. European Journal of Immunology. 2009;**39**:2325–2330. doi: 10.1002/eji.200939548.

[50] Moser M. Dendritic cells in immunity and tolerance-do they display opposite functions? Immunity. 2003;**19**:5–8.

[51] Quah BJ, O'Neill HC. Maturation of function in dendritic cells for tolerance and immunity. Journal of Cellular and Molecular Medicine. 2005;**9**:643–654.

[52] Rescigno M. Dendritic cells in oral tolerance in the gut. Cellular Microbiology. 2011;**13**:1312–1318. doi: 10.1111/j.1462-5822.2011.01626.x.

[53] Steinman RM. Dendritic cells: understanding immunogenicity. European Journal of Immunology. 2007;**37 Suppl 1**:S53-60. doi: 10.1002/eji.200737400.

[54] Steinman RM, Swanson J. The endocytic activity of dendritic cells. Journal of Experimental Medicine. 1995;**182**:283–288.

[55] Platta HW, Stenmark H. Endocytosis and signaling. Current Opinion in Cell Biology. 2011;**23**:393–403.

[56] Sorkin A, von Zastrow M. Endocytosis and signalling: intertwining molecular networks. Nature Reviews Molecular Cell Biology. 2009;**10**:609–622. doi: 10.1038/nrm2748.

[57] Burgdorf S, Kurts C. Endocytosis mechanisms and the cell biology of antigen. Current Opinion in Immunology. 2008;**20**:89–95.

[58] Jensen PE. Recent advances in antigen processing and presentation Nature Immunology. 2007;**8**:1041–1048.

[59] Gallucci S, Matzinger P. Danger signals: SOS to the immune system. Current Opinion in Immunology. 2001;**13**:114–119.

[60] Wagner JG, Roth RA. Neutrophil migration mechanisms, with an emphasis on the pulmonary vasculature. Pharmacological Reviews. 2000;**52**:349–374.

[61] Medzhitov R, Janeway C, Jr. The Toll receptor family and microbial recognition. Trends in Microbiology. 2000;**8**:452–456.

[62] Pulendran B, Ahmed R. Translating innate immunity into immunological memory: Implications for vaccine development. Cell. 2006;**124**:849–863.

[63] Rossi D, Zlotnik A. The biology of chemokines and their receptors. Annual Review of Immunology. 2000;**18**:217–242. doi: 10.1146/annurev.immunol.18.1.217.

[64] Dzopalic T, Rajkovic I, Dragicevic A, Colic M. The response of human dendritic cells to co-ligation of pattern-recognition receptors. Immunologic Research. 2012;**52**:20–33. doi: 10.1007/s12026-012-8279-5.

[65] Ouasti S, Kingham PJ, Terenghi G, Tirelli N. The CD44/integrins interplay and the significance of receptor binding and re-presentation in the uptake of RGD-functionalized hyaluronic acid. Biomaterials. 2011;**33**:1120–34.

[66] van der Goot FG, Gruenberg J. Oiling the wheels of the endocytic pathway. Trends in Cell Biology. 2002;**12**:296–299.

[67] Kaisho T. Pathogen sensors and chemokine receptors in dendritic cell subsets. Vaccine. 2012;**30**:7652–7657. doi: 10.1016/j.vaccine.2012.10.043.

[68] Kawai T, Akira S. Toll-like receptor and RIG-I-like receptor signaling. Annals of the New York Academy of Sciences. 2008;**1143**:1–20. doi: 10.1196/annals.1443.020.

[69] Watts C, West MA, Zaru R. TLR signalling regulated antigen presentation in dendritic cells. Current Opinion in Immunology. 2010;**22**:124–130.

[70] Takeuchi O, Akira S. Innate immunity to virus infection. Immunological Reviews. 2009; **277**:75–86.

[71] Ceppi M, Ruggli N, Tache V, Gerber H, McCullough KC, Summerfield A. Double-stranded secondary structures on mRNA induce type 1 interferon (IFN a/b) production and maturation of mRNA-transfected monocyte-derived dendritic cells. Journal of Gene Medicine. 2005;**7**:452–465.

[72] Martina BE. Dengue pathogenesis: a disease driven by the host response. Science Progress. 2014;**97**:197–214.

[73] Teijaro JR. The role of cytokine responses during influenza virus pathogenesis and potential therapeutic options. Current Topics in Microbiology and Immunology. 2015;**386**:3–22. doi: 10.1007/82_2014_411.

[74] Tisoncik JR, Korth MJ, Simmons CP, Farrar J, Martin TR, Katze MG. Into the eye of the cytokine storm. Microbiology and Molecular Biology Reviews. 2012;**76**:16–32. doi: 10.1128/MMBR.05015-11.

[75] McCullough KC, Ruggli N, Summerfield A. Dendritic cells—at the front-line of pathogen attack. Veterinary Immunology and Immunopathology. 2009;**128**:7–15. doi: 10.1016/j.vetimm.2008.10.290.

[76] Diaz-San Segundo F, Rodriguez-Calvo T, de Avila A, Sevilla N. Immunosuppression during acute infection with foot-and-mouth disease virus in swine is mediated by IL-10. PLoS One. 2009;**4**:e5659. doi: 10.1371/journal.pone.0005659.

[77] Summerfield A, Guzylack-Piriou L, Harwood L, McCullough KC. Innate immune responses against foot-and-mouth disease virus: current understanding and future directions. Veterinary Immunology and Immunopathology. 2009;**128**:205–210. doi: 10.1016/j.vetimm.2008.10.296.

[78] Pelkmans L, Helenius A. Endocytosis via caveolae. Traffic. 2002;**3**:311–320.

[79] Bonifacino JS, Lippincott-Schwartz J. Coat proteins: shaping membrane transport. Nature Reviews Molecular Cell Biology. 2003;**4**:409–414. doi: 10.1038/nrm1099.

[80] Kirchhausen T. Clathrin. Annual Review of Biochemistry. 2000;**69**:699–727. doi: 10.1146/annurev.biochem.69.1.699.

[81] Marsh M, Helenius A. Virus entry: open sesame. Cell. 2006;**124**:729–740. doi: S0092-8674(06)00182-6 [pii], 10.1016/j.cell.2006.02.007.

[82] Rust MJ, Lakadamyali M, Zhang F, Zhuang X. Assembly of endocytic machinery around individual influenza viruses during viral entry. Nature Structural & Molecular Biology. 2004;**11**:567–573. doi: 10.1038/nsmb769, nsmb769 [pii].

[83] Sandvig K, Olsnes S, Brown JE, Petersen OW, van Deurs B. Endocytosis from coated pits of Shiga toxin: a glycolipid-binding protein from Shigella dysenteriae 1. Journal of Cell Biology. 1989;**108**:1331–1343.

[84] Morris RE, Gerstein AS, Bonventre PF, Saelinger CB. Receptor-mediated entry of diphtheria toxin into monkey kidney (Vero) cells: electron microscopic evaluation. Infection and Immunity. 1985;**50**:721–727.

[85] Abrami L, Bischofberger M, Kunz B, Groux R, van der Goot FG. Endocytosis of the anthrax toxin is mediated by clathrin, actin and unconventional adaptors. PLoS Pathogens. 2010;**6**:e1000792. doi: 10.1371/journal.ppat.1000792.

[86] Watts C. Capture and processing of exogenous antigens for presentation on MHC molecules. Annual Review of Immunology. 1997;**15**:821–850. doi: 10.1146/annurev.immunol.15.1.821.

[87] de Baey A, Lanzavecchia A. The role of aquaporins in dendritic cell macropinocytosis. Journal of Experimental Medicine. 2000;**191**:743–748.

[88] Sallusto F, Cella M, Danieli C, Lanzavecchia A. Dendritic cells use macropinocytosis and the mannose receptor to concentrate macromolecules in the major histocompatibility complex class II compartment: downregulation by cytokines and bacterial products. Journal of Experimental Medicine. 1995;**182**:389–400.

[89] Racoosin EL, Swanson JA. Macropinosome maturation and fusion with tubular lysosomes in macrophages. Journal of Cell Biology. 1993;**121**:1011–1020.

[90] Hewlett LJ, Prescott AR, Watts C. The coated pit and macropinocytic pathways serve distinct endosome populations. Journal of Cell Biology. 1994;**124**:689–703.

[91] Schnatwinkel C, Christoforidis S, Lindsay MR, Uttenweiler-Joseph S, Wilm M, Parton RG, Zerial M. The Rab5 effector Rabankyrin-5 regulates and coordinates different endocytic mechanisms. PLoS Biology. 2004;**2**:E261. doi: 10.1371/journal.pbio.0020261.

[92] Lutz MB, Rovere P, Kleijmeer MJ, Rescigno M, Assmann CU, Oorschot VM, Geuze HJ, Trucy J, Demandolx D, Davoust J, Ricciardi-Castagnoli P. Intracellular routes and selective retention of antigens in mildly acidic cathepsin D/lysosome-associated membrane protein-1/MHC class II-positive vesicles in immature dendritic cells. Journal of Immunology. 1997;**159**:3707–3716.

[93] Falnes PO, Sandvig K. Penetration of protein toxins into cells. Current Opinion in Cell Biology. 2000;**12**:407–413. doi: S0955-0674(00)00109-5 [pii].

[94] Lamaze C, Dujeancourt A, Baba T, Lo CG, Benmerah A, Dautry-Varsat A. Interleukin 2 receptors and detergent-resistant membrane domains define a clathrin-independent endocytic pathway. Molecular Cell. 2001;**7**:661–671. doi: S1097-2765(01)00212-X [pii].

[95] Pelkmans L, Burli T, Zerial M, Helenius A. Caveolin-stabilized membrane domains as multifunctional transport and sorting devices in endocytic membrane traffic. Cell. 2004;**118**:767–780. doi: 10.1016/j.cell.2004.09.003, S0092867404008335 [pii].

[96] Schnitzer JE, Oh P, Pinney E, Allard J. Filipin-sensitive caveolae-mediated transport in endothelium: reduced transcytosis, scavenger endocytosis, and capillary permeability of select macromolecules. Journal of Cell Biology. 1994;**127**:1217–1232.

[97] Herreros J, Ng T, Schiavo G. Lipid rafts act as specialized domains for tetanus toxin binding and internalization into neurons. Molecular Biology of the Cell. 2001;12: 2947–2960.

[98] Shogomori H, Futerman AH. Cholera toxin is found in detergent-insoluble rafts/ domains at the cell surface of hippocampal neurons but is internalized via a raft-independent mechanism. Journal of Biological Chemistry. 2001;**276**:9182–9188. doi: 10.1074/jbc.M009414200, M009414200 [pii].

[99] Anderson HA, Chen Y, Norkin LC. Bound simian virus 40 translocates to caveolin-enriched membrane domains, and its entry is inhibited by drugs that selectively disrupt caveolae. Molecular Biology of the Cell. 1996;7:1825–1834.

[100] Lencer WI, Hirst TR, Holmes RK. Membrane traffic and the cellular uptake of cholera toxin. Biochimica et Biophysica Acta. 1999;1450:177–190. doi: S0167-4889(99)00070-1 [pii].

[101] Tran D, Carpentier JL, Sawano F, Gorden P, Orci L. Ligands internalized through coated or noncoated invaginations follow a common intracellular pathway. Proceedings of the National Academy of Sciences of the United States of America. 1987;84:7957–7961.

[102] Orlandi PA, Fishman PH. Filipin-dependent inhibition of cholera toxin: evidence for toxin internalization and activation through caveolae-like domains. Journal of Cell Biology. 1998;141:905–915.

[103] Nichols BJ, Lippincott-Schwartz J. Endocytosis without clathrin coats. Trends in Cell Biology. 2001;11:406–412. doi: S0962-8924(01)02107-9 [pii].

[104] Falguieres T, Mallard F, Baron C, Hanau D, Lingwood C, Goud B, Salamero J, Johannes L. Targeting of Shiga toxin B-subunit to retrograde transport route in association with detergent-resistant membranes. Molecular Biology of the Cell. 2001;12:2453–2468.

[105] Pelkmans L, Kartenbeck J, Helenius A. Caveolar endocytosis of simian virus 40 reveals a new two-step vesicular-transport pathway to the ER. Nature Cell Biology. 2001;3:473–483. doi: 10.1038/35074539.

[106] Midoux P, Pichon C, Yaouanc J-J, Jaffrès P-A. Chemical vectors for gene delivery: a current review on polymers, peptides and lipids containing histidine or imidazole as nucleic acids carriers. British Journal of Pharmacology. 2009;157:166–178.

[107] Varkouhi AK, Scholte M, Storm G, Haisma HJ. Endosomal escape pathways for delivery of biologicals. Journal of Controlled Release. 2011;151:220–228.

[108] Won Y-W, Lim KS, Kim Y-H. Intracellular organelle-targeted non-viral gene delivery systems. Journal of Controlled Release. 2011;152:99–109.

[109] Nakase I, Kobayashi S, Futaki S. Endosome-disruptive peptides for improving cytosolic delivery of bioactive macromolecules. Biopolymers: Peptide Science. 2010;94: 763–770.

[110] Wasungu L, Hoekstra D. Cationic lipids, lipoplexes and intracellular delivery of genes. Journal of Controlled Release. 2006;116:255–264.

[111] Vyas JM, Van der Veen AG, Ploegh HL. The known unknowns of antigen processing and presentation. Nature Reviews Immunology. 2008;8:607–618.

[112] Belizaire R, Unanue ER. Targeting proteins to distinct subcellular compartments reveals unique requirements for MHC class I and II presentation. Proceedings of the National Academy of Sciences. 2009;106:17463–17468.

[113] Neefjes J, Jongsma ML, Paul P, Bakke O. Towards a systems understanding of MHC class I and MHC class II antigen presentation. Nature Reviews Immunology. 2011;11:823–836. doi: 10.1038/nri3084.

[114] McCullough KC, Milona P, Démoulins T, Englezou P, Ruggli N. Dendritic Cell Targets for Self-Replicating RNA Vaccines. Journal of Blood and Lymph. 2015;5:132. epub 10.4172/2165-7831.1000132. doi: 10.4172/2165-7831.1000132.

[115] Atkins GJ, Fleeton MN, Sheahan BJ. Therapeutic and prophylactic applications of alphavirus vectors. Expert Reviews in Molecular Medicine. 2008;10:e33. doi: 10.1017/S1462399408000859.

[116] Khromykh AA. Replicon-based vectors of positive strand RNA viruses. Current Opinion in Molecular Therapy. 2000;2:555–569.

[117] Rayner JO, Dryga SA, Kamrud KI. Alphavirus vectors and vaccination. Reviews in Medical Virology. 2002;12:279–296. doi: 10.1002/rmv.360.

[118] Suter R, Summerfield A, Thomann-Harwood LJ, McCullough KC, Tratschin JD, Ruggli N. Immunogenic and replicative properties of classical swine fever virus replicon particles modified to induce IFN-alpha/beta and carry foreign genes. Vaccine. 2011;29:1491–1503. doi: 10.1016/j.vaccine.2010.12.026.

[119] Lundstrom K. Alphavirus-based vaccines. Current Opinion in Molecular Therapy. 2002;4:28–34.

[120] Pijlman GP, Suhrbier A, Khromykh AA. Kunjin virus replicons: an RNA-based, non-cytopathic viral vector system for protein production, vaccine and gene therapy applications. Expert Opinion on Biological Therapy. 2006;6:135–145. doi: 10.1517/14712598.6.2.135.

[121] Ljungberg K, Liljestrom P. Self-replicating alphavirus RNA vaccines. Expert Review Vaccines. 2015;14:177–194. doi: 10.1586/14760584.2015.965690.

[122] McCullough KC. Combatting disease. pan European networks: Science and Technology. 2014;**11**:168–169.

[123] Demoulins T, Bassi I, Thomann-Harwood L, Jandus C, Kaeuper P, Simon HU, von Gunten S, McCullough KC. Alginate-coated chitosan nanogel capacity to modulate the effect of TLR ligands on blood dendritic cells. Nanomedicine. 2013;9:806–817. doi: 10.1016/j.nano.2013.01.002.

Chapter 6

Myelomonocytic Cell Lines in Modeling HIV-1 Infection of the Bone Marrow

Michael R. Nonnemacher, Shane Quiterio, Alexander G. Allen, Anthony R. Mele, Vanessa Pirrone and Brian Wigdahl

Additional information is available at the end of the chapter

http://dx.doi.org/10.5772/67596

Abstract

Human immunodeficiency virus type 1 (HIV-1), the etiologic agent of acquired immunodeficiency syndrome (AIDS), primarily infects T cells and cells of the monocyte-macrophage lineage. This is due to the presence of the cell surface receptor CD4 and the coreceptors, CXCR4, and CCR5. While the T-cell has classically been the cell type associated with HIV-1 disease progression, cells of the monocyte-macrophage lineage have also been shown to play a major role in this viral pathologic process. Classically, this has involved monocytic cells in the peripheral blood and tissue macrophages, however, over the course of HIV disease, the promyelomonocytic cells of the bone marrow (BM) have also been shown to play a role in pathogenesis retroviral disease in that they play an integral role in the reseeding of the periphery and end-organ tissues. This has involved an initial infection of the bone marrow hematopoietic progenitor cells. Given this observation, over the years there have been a number of cell lines that have been developed and provided valuable insights into research questions surrounding HIV-1 infection of the monocyte-macrophage cell lineage. In this regard, we will examine the biological and immunological properties of these BM-derived cell lines with respect to their utility in exploring the pathogenesis of HIV-1 in humans.

Keywords: HIV-1, HL-60, TF-1, myelomonocytic cells, latency

1. Introduction

Human immunodeficiency virus type 1 (HIV-1) has been shown to primarily infect cells of the lymphoid and myeloid lineages in the peripheral blood and bone marrow (BM). One of the roles of the bone marrow serves to repopulate the peripheral blood with fresh circulating cells in response to stimuli. During HIV-1 disease, the BM has been shown to be dysfunctional leading to the pathology commonly observed in the acquired immunodeficiency syndrome (AIDS), with thrombocytopenia, anemia, monocytopenia, and neutrocytopenia [1, 2]. HIV-1 infection of bone marrow stromal cells, changes in the cytokine milieu of the bone marrow, and cytotoxic effects of HIV-1 proteins are pathogenic mechanisms involved in the impairment of the differentiation and growth of hematopoietic progenitor cells (HPCs), ultimately leading to hematopoietic defects [3–5] during the course of HIV disease. Interestingly, HIV-1 DNA was not detected in bone marrow–derived CD34$^+$ HPCs in HIV-1–infected patients on combination antiretroviral [6]. However, other investigators have detected HIV-1 DNA in CD34$^+$ HPCs in patients who are on antiretroviral therapy [7]. Numerous coinfections, as well as some lymphomas commonly observed in AIDS patients [8], have been shown to further impact hematopoiesis in HIV-1–infected individuals. Direct HIV-1 infection of hematopoietic progenitor cells may contribute to hematopoietic abnormalities; however, the extent of infection in the bone marrow compartment remains controversial [9]. Numerous studies have demonstrated the susceptibility of CD34$^+$ bone marrow–derived cell populations to HIV-1 both *in vivo* and *in vitro* [10–13]. In general, the permittivity of CD34$^+$ HPCs has been shown to depend on the state of differentiation, with the committed progenitor cells being the most susceptible and the quiescent stem cells being the most refractile to HIV-1 infection [14, 15]. In this regard, it has been shown that macrophage colony stimulating factor (M-CSF) [11] induces HIV-1 infection of HPCs and subsequent virus production involving increased CD4 expression and enhanced viral replicative processes, respectively, emphasizing the crucial role that physiological changes in the bone marrow environment have on the HIV-1 susceptibility replicative capabilities of this cellular compartment.

During the course of chronic HIV-1 infection, there is a characteristic loss of CD4$^+$ T cells over time in the absence of effective therapy. However, with the era of highly active antiretroviral therapy (HAART), this trend has been reversed. Interestingly, over the course of this time, cells of the myeloid lineage, even though CD4$^+$, have been shown to less susceptible to virus-induced cytopathic effect and cell death with a drop in cell numbers much less evident during disease progression [16]. In addition, this cell lineage has been shown to be able to traverse various endothelial cell barriers, including the blood-brain barrier, allowing the infected circulating cell of the monocytic lineage to transport HIV into tissues as perivascular macrophages [17, 18]. Once in tissues, the emerging infectious HIV-1 particle can then go on to infect other resident cells of that tissue. As these cells migrate to other tissues and as the immune response causes a general state of inflammation, the bone marrow is involving in replacing cells lost to infection and to facilitate the immunologic response to HIV infection. Given that there are reports of HPCs becoming infected in the bone marrow, one intriguing possibility is that mature progenitor cells or cells that are committed to the monocyte lineage but still capable of a limited number of cell divisions, may be infected by HIV-1 while still in the bone marrow and subsequently migrate to the blood and subsequently into peripheral tissues thereby contributing to the continued viral dissemination [19].

Given these observations, we will briefly review hematopoiesis to define how myeloid cells differentiate from hematopoietic stem cells (HSCs). We will then review the literature that

http://dx.doi.org/10.5772/67596

demonstrates the bone marrow as a site of HIV-1 infection. This approach will provide a framework to review and assess the literature concerning a number of cell lines that are currently available to be used to model virus-host interactions, as well as experimental paradigms that have utilized these cell lines to understand basic virologic and immunologic concepts relevant to HIV infection. Finally, it will conclude by discussing the next most important pressing experiments to be performed and what questions these experiments will answer to understand HIV-1 infection of the bone marrow compartment and myeloid lineage of cells.

2. $CD34^+$ hematopoietic stem and progenitor cells

All cells of the hematopoietic system are derived from a common precursor cell, the hematopoietic stem cell (**Figure 1**) [20]. Stem cells are defined as single cells that are clonal precursors of more stem cells of the same type, as well as a defined set of differentiated progeny cells [20, 21]. Stem cells normally represent only about 0.05% of cells in the bone marrow, and their population is maintained at a constant level through self-renewal [22]. $CD34^+$ progenitor cell populations, which are heterogeneous cell population containing true pluripotent stem cells and other more mature cells, are often used for hematopoietic stem cell transplantation [23]. The ability of the hematopoietic stem cells to home to the bone marrow following intravenous injection is mediated by the interactions of selectins on bone marrow endothelial cells with integrins on the

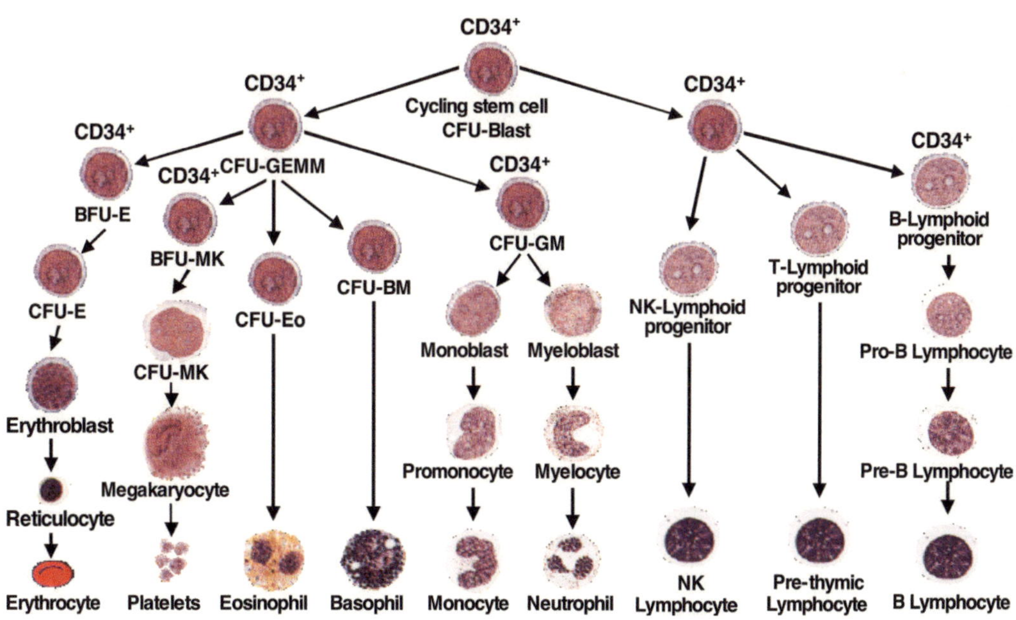

Figure 1. Differentiation of $CD34^+$ stem cells. $CD34^+$ stem cells can be differentiated into all of the cell types that are found in the blood. Cells have to go through a number of differentiated stages of progenitor and immature cells to finally become a mature blood cell. As a cell differentiates it commits to numerous cell lineages. Adapted from Ref. [31].

hematopoietic cells [24]. The CD34 sialomucin receptor is one of the several adhesions involved in the intra and extramedullary homing of progenitor cells into distinct microenvironments [25, 26]. The CD34 antigen is expressed on primitive human hematopoietic cells capable of both self-renewal and differentiation into diverse blood cell lineages [27]. HPCs normally reside in the bone marrow in close contact with the cells of stroma that provide cytokines, extracellular matrix proteins, and adhesion molecules [28]. Progenitor cells are compartmentalized in different areas of the bone marrow based on their degree of commitment and lineage differentiation [29]. Bone marrow–derived $CD34^+$ cells isolated from HIV-1–infected individuals have a diminished colony potential [30]. Studying infection of $CD34^+$ progenitor cells is important in understanding the cytopenias and impaired colony growth in advanced stage HIV-1–infected patients [8].

$CD34^+$ cells are a heterogeneous population of multipotent hematopoietic progenitors at different stages of differentiation, residing in the adult bone marrow [32]. The $CD34^+CD38^-$ immunophenotype defines a rare, quiescent (when a cell is neither dividing nor preparing to divide, remaining in the G_0 cell phase) subpopulation of primitive progenitor cells than can be functionally distinguished from committed $CD34^+/CD38^+$ progenitor cells by sustained clonogenicity in a long-term culture [33]. The more primitive $CD34^+CD38^-$ cells are resistant to infection while the more committed $CD34^+CD38^+$ cells are more susceptible to HIV-1 infection [14]. Primitive hematopoietic cells are not directly infected though their function is markedly disturbed by the presence of virus [34]. HIV-1–infected individuals have been shown to have a decrease in the fraction of $CD34^+/CD38^-$ stem cells in the bone marrow, compared to the healthy individuals [35]. No CD4 expression was detectable on the more primitive $CD34^+CD38^-$ cells and no evidence for infection of these cells was demonstrated [14].

Hematopoietic stem cells are characterized by an extensive capacity for proliferation and differentiation, as well as the ability to self-renew. Stem cells give rise to daughter cells, which undergo irreversible differentiation along a number of different hematopoietic cell lineages [36]. Hematopoiesis consists of a cascade of finely regulated events by which totipotent stem cells differentiate to all cells present in the blood [37]. Lineage commitment, differentiation, maturation, and release of cells into the blood are under the control of a number of hematopoietic growth factors. Differentiation of hematopoietic stem and progenitor cells involves a series of molecular changes that result in progressive loss of self-renewal ability and pluripotency, and in parallel acquisition of specialized functions characteristic of mature blood cells [38]. Stem cells undergo two sequential differentiating processes; the first is commitment, by which stem cells lose their self-renewing capability and differentiate to other cells with a more limited differentiating potential. The second process is maturation, which allows the terminal differentiation of those cells committed to a specific terminal lineage [39]. Both the commitment and the maturation of hematopoietic cells arise from the gradual expression of lineage-specific genes. Commitment is defined as the decision a cell makes to enter, or generate progeny that enters, a particular maturation lineage at some future time [36]. This decision does not necessarily have to be accompanied by any immediate change in morphology or expression of novel membrane proteins or regulator receptors. Hematopoietic commitment is likely to be extrinsically regulated, but there is only limited evidence, and probably only a limited opportunity, for hematopoietic regulators to be involved in the commitment events [36]. Once established, maturation programs do not seem to be qualitatively altered by the particular growth factors that activate mature cell production [36]. Most of the cell differentiation pathway takes place in the bone marrow. As CD34⁺ cells differentiate, they can commit to a specific lineage at specifically defined branch points (**Figure 1**). A number of cytokines influence and promote the cell differentiation process. Once the cells have differentiated to monocytes, they can travel through the blood and migrate into tissues where they can become tissue macrophages or dendritic cells (**Figure 2**).

3. Cells of the monocyte-macrophage lineage

Monocytes belong to the mononuclear phagocytic system and constitute 3–8% of the peripheral blood leukocytes. Monocytic nuclei are eccentric, either oval or kidney shaped and contain small vacuoles in the cytoplasm that are lysosomes filled with degradative enzymes. Monocytes originate from promonocytes, which are rapidly dividing precursors in the bone marrow. When the mature cells enter the peripheral blood, they are termed monocytes (**Figure 2**). The monocytes often leave the blood and infiltrate tissues, undergoing additional changes and are then referred to as macrophages [40]. Macrophages act as effector cells, attacking microorganisms and neoplastic cells and removing foreign material, as well as presenting antigen

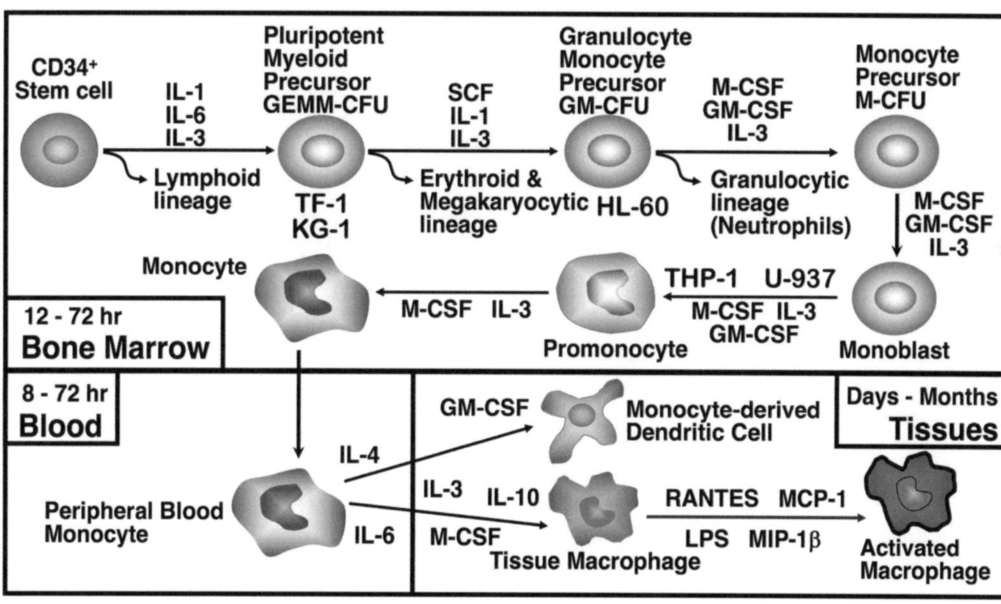

Figure 2. Differentiation of monocytes-macrophages from CD34⁺ stem cells. The monocytic differentiation pathway and growth factors are involved, as well as the sites where the differentiation takes place is depicted. The majority of the cell differentiation stages occur within the bone marrow. As the CD34+ cell differentiates, it commits to the myeloid lineage at various branch points for other lineages, such as the lymphoid, erythroid, and granulocytic lineages. A number of cytokines that influence and promote cell differentiation are also shown. Certain cell lines and the point at which they are located in the cell differentiation pathway are also indicated. Once the cells have differentiated into monocytes, they can travel through the blood and migrate into tissues where they can become tissue macrophages or dendritic cells and also be activated.

to lymphocytes [41]. Macrophages contain receptors for antibody and complement, which enhance their ability to phagocytose organisms. Macrophages produce an enormous number of soluble factors that are important in the immune response and in the process of inflammation.

Monocytic cells are generated in the bone marrow from pluripotent stem cells that can differentiate into multiple hematologic cell types. Within the bone marrow, cytokines induce stem cells to divide and to produce lineages committed to differentiating into monocytic, granulocytic, erythroid, or megakaryocytic cell types (**Figure 2**) [42, 43]. The pluripotent progenitor cell, called the granulocyte-erythroid-megakaryocyte-macrophage colony forming unit (GEMM-CFU), becomes further committed toward either the granulocytic or monocytic phenotype in the presence of IL-1 and/or IL-3, becoming the granulocyte-macrophage colony forming unit (GM-CFU) (**Figure 2**) [39, 42, 43]. The granulocytic and monocytic lineages are closely bound together throughout hematopoiesis and are commonly referred to as the myelomonocytic lineage [42, 43]. Repopulation of the myelomonocytic GM-CFU occurs in the presence of IL-3 or granulocyte-macrophage colony stimulating factor (GM-CSF) [37]. Commitment toward the macrophage lineage requires the presence of macrophage colony stimulating factor (M-CSF), along with IL-3 or GM-CSF [44, 45]. The committed promonocytic cells mature into smaller monocytic cells that can enter the blood. Monocytes circulate within the blood for 8–72 hours before migrating into a number of different tissues where they complete their development, becoming mature tissue macrophages (**Figure 2**) [46–48]. Macrophages are larger in diameter than monocytes and possess increased lysosomal content and hydrolytic enzymes [49]. Macrophages are capable of division and can be a self-sustaining population.

The phenotype and function of the macrophage is dependent on the tissue in which it resides. Therefore, resident macrophages are often defined by the tissue-specific environment in which they ultimately reside. Specific types of macrophages include: the microglial cells of the brain, the Kupffer cells in the liver, the Langerhans cells of the skin, the alveolar macrophages of the lung, the mesangial cells of the kidney, and the sinus macrophages of the spleen [50–52].

4. Bone marrow hematopoiesis disorders associated with HIV-1 infection

Hematologic abnormalities are very common in HIV-1–infected individuals and they occur at all stages of disease, but the mechanisms by which HIV-1 contributes to these abnormalities are poorly understood [53, 54]. HIV-1 affects the hematopoietic system, causing a number of peripheral blood cytopenias [55, 56]. HIV-1–infected patients suffer from many hematologic disorders and exhibit uni or multilineage suppression of bone marrow hematopoiesis including anemia, lymphocytopenia, thrombocytopenia, granulocytopenia, monocytopenia, and neutropenia that can be attributed to malfunction or premature death of the specific hematopoietic cells [8, 57–59]. The hematopoietic disorders are frequently associated with impaired HPC growth, BM dysplasia, plasmacytosis, and lymphoid infiltrates [57, 60], and they suggest virus-induced abnormalities in the bone marrow microenvironment [61–63]. T cell depletion in AIDS is thought to be, at least in part, due to the failure of T cell development from lymphohematopoietic stem cells [14].

A large number of studies have been conducted to identify and characterize the pathophysiologic mechanisms leading to bone marrow dysfunction in patients with AIDS. HIV-1 may affect hematopoietic stem cells (HSCs) by both direct and indirect mechanisms leading to defects in maturation of CD34$^+$ cells and the numerous cytopenias. A number of indirect mechanisms for HIV-1–induced suppression of hematopoiesis have been proposed, such as: the stimulation of abnormal cytokine production by HIV-1 infection [30, 64], the suppressive effects of viral gene products [65, 66], and the activation of apoptosis by gp120-mediated cross-linking of CD4 [67]. Hematologic abnormalities in the majority of infected individuals could result from indirect effects of HIV-1, such as cytokine dysregulation, rather than HIV-1 expression in the bone marrow itself [53]. HIV-1 Tat has been shown to decrease differentiation in an HPC line [68]. In addition, the viral accessory protein Nef has been shown to decrease hematopoiesis *in vitro* [69]. Studies have also demonstrated that HIV-1 may induce apoptosis in hematopoietic cell lines [70, 71]. Modification of the behavior of hematopoietic accessory cells by HIV-1 infection may indirectly alter the growth and differentiation of adjacent uninfected lymphoid, myeloid, and primitive hematopoietic cell populations and account for HIV-1–mediated suppression of hematopoiesis [72]. Infection of auxiliary cells, particular macrophages, and microvascular endothelial cells, induces a substantial alteration in the supportive function of the hematopoietic stromal tissues, indirectly influencing the survival and growth of hematopoietic progenitors [8].

5. Role of growth factors, cytokines, and cellular activation in HIV-1 pathogenesis in the bone marrow

Stem cells, progenitor populations, and their progeny are largely defined by their cytokine responsiveness and cytokine receptor phenotype. Cytokines are soluble glycoproteins that act through cell surface receptors at very low concentrations and control the production of stem cells. The most prominent cytokines are erythropoietin for the production of red blood cells, GM-CSF for granulocytes and macrophages, G-CSF for granulocytes, thrombopoietin for platelets, and M-CSF or CSF-1 for monocyte-macrophage production and function. Cytokines may be stimulatory or inhibitory and may show additive or synergistic effects on the renewal, proliferation, survival, and differentiation of cells. They can also modulate cell migration and adherence. Cytokines are important components of the immunoregulatory network and have been demonstrated to play a major role in the regulation of HIV-1 expression *in vitro*. Potent modulation of HIV-1 expression has been demonstrated either by manipulating endogenous cytokines or by adding exogenous cytokines to culture. The net level of virus replication in an HIV-1–infected individual reflects, in part, the balance between inductive and suppressive host factors that are mediated mainly by cytokines. Reverse transcription, integration, and virus spread are much more efficient in cells that have been activated by cytokines.

Cytokines and growth factors function by activating a number of different transcription factors. Sequentially ordered activation of transcription factors controls lineage commitment. Once a particular set of transcription factors has been induced, reversibility is limited. In the early phases of differentiation, the regulatory roles of the growth factors overlap [36]. Later in development, some growth factors are lineage-specific, and govern the maturation of single lineages. Hematopoietic cells have distinctive patterns of growth factor receptor expression that evolve as the cells differentiate [36]. Binding of the growth factors to their receptors leads to activation of intracellular kinases and triggers cell proliferation [73, 74]. Hematopoietic growth factors not only stimulate cell proliferation, but also prolong cell survival by exhibiting antiapoptotic effects. Growth factors, such as G-CSF and GM-CSF, can stimulate early hematopoietic cell proliferation, increase the number of cells produced by the bone marrow, prolong the life span of cells, and augment cell function [75]. In the marrow, blood cells develop in two phases: the proliferative and the maturational phases. During cell proliferation, the precursors of blood cells normally undergo cell division at intervals of about 18–24 hours. In the maturational phase, cell division ceases, but additional modifications occur before the cell enters the blood. Progenitor cells exhibit a higher proliferative rate and more lineage restriction than stem cells. They are also responsive to a smaller subset of cytokines. The production of all cell types is controlled by a negative feedback mechanism. When demand for specific cell types increases, or peripheral levels of the cells fall, then stimulatory cytokines are released to generate new cells within a few days.

6. Organization of bone marrow and its role as a viral reservoir

Hematopoietic cells develop within the medullary space, which has a rich vascular supply and is populated by many cell types including: adipocytes, vascular endothelial cells, fibroblasts, and stromal cells (**Figure 3**). The frequency of HSCs in the bone marrow is relatively constant [76, 77]. Vascular endothelial cells, marrow fibroblasts, and stromal cells produce hematopoietic growth factors and chemokines that regulate blood cell production [78]. Vascular endothelial cells form a barrier that keeps immature cells in the marrow and permits mature cells to enter the blood. Macrophages in the bone marrow remove dead or apoptotic cells and clear the blood of foreign materials that enter the marrow (**Figure 3**). Stem cells and primitive cells bind tightly to the stroma, while maturing precursors and terminally differentiated cells are nonadherent.

The bone marrow may serve as an important reservoir of HIV-1 in the body. Previous results have suggested that the bone marrow macrophages may act as a reservoir for HIV, and infection of this cell population may affect hematopoiesis, either by transmission of HIV infection to developing progenitor cells or by altering the ability of the stroma to support normal development [80]. The circulating $CD34^+$ progenitor cell population may be infected *in vivo* and may serve as a reservoir for HIV-1 that is capable of trafficking the virus to diverse anatomic compartments [13]. Peripheral blood–derived $CD34^+$ progenitor cells may also be infected and disseminate HIV-1 to sites throughout the body. Integration of proviral DNA into stem cell genomes could lead to the spread of HIV-1 infection through the expansion of infected clones or interference with normal stem cell maturation and proliferation, resulting in the interruption of normal hematopoiesis [14]. Studies have shown that primary $CD34^+$ progenitor cells are susceptible to infection by diverse strains of HIV-1, particularly as they begin to differentiate, and infection can be sustained for prolonged periods *in vitro* [13, 32]. This may contribute to a chronically infected pool of functionally altered cells containing viruses of different tropism across different cell lineages [32].

http://dx.doi.org/10.5772/67596

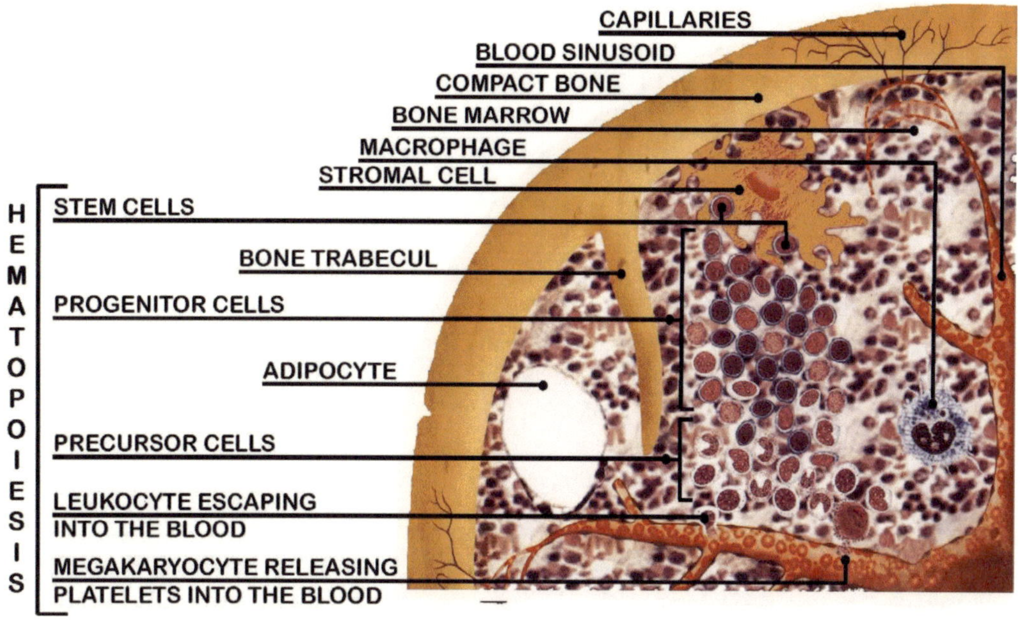

Figure 3. Hematopoiesis within the bone marrow. Hematopoiesis occurs within the bone marrow and begins with stem cells associated with stromal cells that nourish them and supply growth factors. Stem cells differentiate through various stages of progenitor cells and commit to various cell lineages eventually entering the blood circulation. Adapted from Ref. [79].

7. Direct infection of CD34⁺ hematopoietic progenitor cells by HIV-1

Direct involvement of HIV-1 infection may be important in leading to HSC failure and bone marrow dysfunction [59]. Direct infection and destruction of hematopoietic stem or progenitor cells may explain the defective hematopoiesis in HIV-1–infected individuals [81]. Attempts to understand HIV-1–mediated bone marrow dysfunction have yielded inconsistent results regarding the susceptibility of bone marrow progenitors to viral infection [14]. Conflicting studies have been reported regarding the susceptibility of human $CD34^+$ cells to HIV-1 infection both *in vivo* and *in vitro*, and there has been a significant controversy regarding whether HIV-1 can infect HSCs directly, leading to bone marrow dysfunction and the cytopenias. A number of studies of HIV-1–infected individuals have failed to detect productively infected $CD34^+$ progenitor cells from the bone marrow [54, 82, 83], while other studies have shown that rare infection of $CD34^+$ progenitor cells can occur [84, 85] and may be more prevalent in patients with advanced disease [86].

Direct infection of the primitive progenitor cells, which represent 0.01% of bone marrow cells, is difficult to detect [13]. Several reports have described that bone marrow $CD34^+$ stem and/or progenitor cells are infected with HIV-1 at low frequencies in some patients [84]. Purified $CD34^+$ HPCs from adult peripheral blood were reported to be susceptible to HIV-1 infection, as shown by PCR analysis for the presence of proviral sequences in the ensuing myeloid and erythroid colonies or by virus production in culture [13, 81, 87]. Several studies have shown successful *in vitro* infection of the $CD34^+$ population [11, 88], although studies in this area have focused on hematological consequences of HIV-1 infection and its effects on progenitor cells [10, 81, 88]. HIV-1 infection *in vitro* has been reported in highly purified bone marrow–derived $CD34^+$ cells [89] and in $CD34^+$ progenitor cells that coexpress CD4 [70]. Based on a number of reports, it was found that a low fraction of progenitor cells is able to be infected *ex vivo* by HIV-1 under certain conditions, the growth of the few cells infected by HIV-1 may not be impaired as a result of the infection, while *in vivo* infection of progenitor cells occurs rarely, if ever [8].

The number of HIV-positive HPCs may sharply increase in advanced AIDS because of widespread HIV-1 infection, thus explaining the reports on *in vivo* HIV-positive $CD34^+$ cells in the advanced disease [85, 86]. Studies suggest that HIV-1-expressing cells are present in the bone marrow during late stages of disease [53]. In individuals with advanced HIV-1 infection, about 1 in 500 $CD34^+$ cells were shown to be infected with HIV-1 [86]. The CFU capacity of the bone marrow stem cells was impaired especially in patients with advanced disease, even if HIV-1 does not directly infect these cells [90]. Depletion of primitive progenitors observed in later stages of HIV-1 disease may represent a virus-induced alteration in progenitor cell differentiation [91–93].

Multiple and potentially synergistic mechanisms may be responsible for the resistance of $CD34^+$ cells to HIV-1 infection [28]. Most studies indicate that bone marrow–derived HSCs cannot be infected by HIV-1 until they undergo modest differentiation in order to express the appropriate receptors to enable virus entry and subsequent replication [59]. Studies have demonstrated the presence of both CD4 [94] and the chemokine receptors CXCR4 and CCR5 [95] on $CD34^+$ cells. The most primitive bone marrow HPCs lack the surface molecules CD4, CXCR4, and CCR5, which are required for HIV-1 infection, so they cannot be infected with HIV-1 [14]. $CD4^+$ cells were found only within the more mature $CD34^+CD38^+$ cell population, explaining their susceptibility to infection [14]. Cell surface expression of CXCR4 and CCR5 has been found on peripheral blood–derived $CD34^+$ progenitor cells [13]. When CD4 expression is low, infection becomes dependent on coreceptor expression levels. High chemokine receptor levels can compensate for low surface expression of CD4 in mediating HIV-1 infection [13]. T-tropic strains of HIV-1 have been shown to infect cultures of purified $CD34^+$ progenitor cells *in vitro*, suggesting the presence of the CXCR4 coreceptor on the cells [62, 81]. The natural chemokine ligands for the major HIV-1 coreceptors are able to readily block entry of HIV-1 [96]. The CC-chemokines RANTES, MIP-1α, and MIP-1β are the natural ligands for CCR5 and block the entry of R5 viruses, whereas SDF-1, the natural ligand for CXCR4, blocks the entry of X4 viruses, thus inhibiting the infection and spread of the virus. The mechanisms relevant to inhibition of HIV-1 infection involve the blocking of binding of the virus to its coreceptor, thus blocking viral entry.

8. Specific viral populations within the CNS suggest bone marrow origination

Because the CNS has been shown to be more "immunologically privileged" than many other organs, it has been suggested that virus enters the CNS early after primary infection and then replicates there beyond the control of the peripheral immune system to a great degree.

http://dx.doi.org/10.5772/67596

In addition, some antiretroviral drugs such as protease inhibitors have trouble crossing the blood-brain barrier [97, 98]. Inefficient drug delivery combined with an "immunologically privileged" site leads to viral reservoirs remaining in the CNS throughout the duration of infection. Viral genome sequence analysis supports the notion that CNS-specific or neurotropic forms of virus exist [99–103]. Recent studies demonstrate that viral sequences within specific CNS regions match, phylogenetically, with sequences found in the bone marrow [104, 105]. This supports the hypothesis that virus could be transported into the CNS in hematogenous-derived cells.

HIV-1 gp160 sequences from postmortem tissues collected from a patient with HIV-1 dementia were isolated and analyzed for sequence similarity [105]. Gartner and colleagues found that the gp160 sequences from patients with dementia demonstrate remarkable sequence similarity between isolates from subcortical regions of the brain (particularly in deep white matter (DWM)) and those of the bone marrow [104]. Phylogenetic analysis showed that the sequences from DWM were more closely related to those from bone marrow and peripheral blood monocytes. Sequences from DWM and monocytes clustered together, indicating greater homology between the HIV-1 species in these groups, as well as a more recent evolutionary divergence between them, relative to the species in other tissues. The phylogenetic tree showed that the bone marrow sequences were clustered with the DWM and monocyte group, although the bone marrow species diverged at an earlier time. Viral species from the DWM were more closely related to those in bone marrow than those in other tissues, with the DWM, monocyte, and bone marrow sequences clustering together as a group. These observations suggest that of bone marrow–derived monocytes traffic into the DWM of the brain during late stage infection. Bone marrow–derived monocytes within the circulation may enter the DWM and become perivascular macrophages, potentially transmitting HIV-1 to neighboring cells [106]. A critical step toward the development of HIV-associate dementia may be an increase in monocyte trafficking into the brain [107]. This process may be either initiated and/or accelerated during late-stage infection, which could explain why dementia occurs at this time. These observations point to the bone marrow as the likely source of virus entering the CNS in terminal stages. The frequency and extent of infection and the kinetics of virus replication in bone marrow are not well classified.

9. Cell lines to model HIV infection of bone marrow

A number of different monocytic progenitor cell lines have been derived that can be used as experimental tools (**Figure 2**). These cell lines will be discussed from the least differentiated to the most differentiated cellular phenotype.

9.1. KG-1

The KG-1 cell line is a $CD34^+/CD38^+$ myelomonocytic progenitor cell line that was derived from the bone marrow of a patient with acute myelogenous leukemia [108]. A variant $CD34^+/CD38^-$ cell line, called the KG-1a subline, morphologically and histochemically resembles undifferentiated blast cells. The KG-1 cell line is composed predominantly of myeloblasts and promyelocytes [109]. KG-1 cells can be induced to differentiate into dendritic-like cells by the addition of GM-CSF and TNF-α, or phorbol 12-myristate 13-acetate (PMA) with ionomycin or TNF-α [110]. KG-1 cells can be induced to differentiate into macrophage-like cells in response to phorbol esters such as 12-O-tetradecanoylphorbol-13-acetate (TPA), while the KG-1a cells are resistant to the effects of TPA [111, 112]. With respect to studies of HIV-1 pathogenesis and disease, this cell line has not been as widely used as you will see for HL-60 and TF-1 cell lines due to a very low to no expression of CD4 on the cell surface [113, 114]. However, many researchers who examine regulation of CD4, CCR5, and CXCR4 on the myeloid cell lineage use this cell line in combination with HL-60, TF-1, and others. Interestingly, a number of studies have examined coinfection of human herpesvirus type 6 (HHV6) and HIV-1 and demonstrated that if KG-1 cells were first infected with HHV6, this would induce CD4 expression thereby facilitating subsequent HIV-1 infection by viruses that use either CCR5 or CXCR4 as the coreceptor [113–115]. They have also been used for studies surrounding toxicity of drugs [116] or for alteration of normal cell function [117] for bone marrow myeloid lineage of cells potentially to be used for HIV treatments.

9.2. TF-1

The TF-1 cell line was established by Kitamura and colleagues in 1987 from a bone marrow aspiration sample of a 35 year old Japanese male with erythroleukemia and severe pancytopenia [118]. TF-1 cells, which have been shown to express several erythroid and myeloid markers, are $CD34^{+}/CD38^{+}$ erythro-myeloid HPCs blocked at an early stage of hematopoietic differentiation [118, 119]. The cells have also been shown to be completely dependent on IL-3 or GM-CSF for long-term growth [118]. Erythropoietin (EPO) also sustains the short-term growth of TF-1 cells but does not induce erythroid differentiation [119]. TF-1 cells can be induced to differentiate into two different pathways, and, depending on the type of inducer, are capable of differentiating into either mature erythroid cells or macrophage-like cells [118]. Hemin and δ-aminolevulinic acid can induce erythroid differentiation with hemoglobin synthesis in TF-1 cells, while PMA induces dramatic differentiation into macrophage-like cells [118]. TF-1 cells consist of a relatively homogenous population of medium-sized cells with the appearance of blasts [120]. They contain moderate amounts of dark basophilic, agranular cytoplasm with frequent small cytoplasmic vacuoles, and have a smooth cytoplasmic border. The nuclei are oval with fine chromatin and 1–3 macronucleoli. Many binucleated and occasional multinucleated forms are present [120].

The TF-1 cell line has provided a useful tool and *in vitro* model system to examine HIV-1 infection of a progenitor cell population during differentiation into monocytic cells. Previous studies have demonstrated that TF-1 cells can be productively infected by the R5-dependent BAL and YU-2 strains of HIV-1, but not by the X4-dependent LAI HIV-1 strain [121]. Differentiation of TF-1 cells down the myeloid pathway or the presence of higher levels of the CCR5 coreceptor as compared to the CXCR4 coreceptor could explain why a productive HIV-1 infection only occurred in cells infected with HIV-1 R5-dependent strains. PMA-induced macrophage-like differentiation of TF-1 cells, characterized by a decrease in nuclear size, an increase in the amount of nuclear chromatin condensation, absence of nucleoli, and increased cytoplasm [120]. The majority of the cells have moderately abundant light basophilic, agranular to finely granular cytoplasm with irregular cytoplasmic borders [120].

TF-1 cells have been used extensively to understand host pathogen interactions between the HIV-1 protein Nef and numerous cellular pathways [122, 123]. These studies have led to a further understanding of how replication is differed between cell types. Specifically, these studies helped identify factors such as STAT3 that are affected by Nef and allow for the survival of TF-1 cells [124]. Like with KG-1 cells, TF-1 cells were also used to confirm that human herpesvirus 6 coinfection with HIV can lead to susceptibility of TF-1 cells to HIV-1 infection [113, 114]. In addition, it was shown in TF-1 cells that lymphocyte function-associated antigen 1 (LFA-1) was needed to confer susceptibility to HIV-1 infection [125]. TF-1 cells have also been used to assess transcriptional activation of the HIV-1 LTR in a number of activation and differentiation states of these cells. This demonstrated the importance of the C/EBP transcription factor in CD34+ progenitor cells for driving LTR activation [126]. In addition, the transcription factors NF-κB and Sp were shown to be important when TF-1 cells were activated by phorbol 12-myristate 13-acetate (PMA), conditioned medium from PMA-treated TF-1 cells, or IL-1² [127, 128].

9.3. HL-60

The HL-60 cell line, obtained by leukapheresis from the peripheral blood of a patient with acute promyelocytic leukemia, is a promyelocytic cell line [129]. In culture, the cells can be stained as promyelocytes or myeloblasts, although only about 10% of the cell population can progress to more mature cells [130]. Differentiation can be induced by a number of agents such as dimethyl sulfoxide (DMSO), butyrate, hypoxanthine, PMA, actinomycin D, and retinoic acid. The cells have the ability to differentiate into either granulocytic or monocytic cells, depending on whether they are treated with either DMSO or PMA, respectively [131–133]. Monocytic differentiation can also be induced by treatment with 1-25 dihydroxyvitamin D_3 or lymphokine [134, 135]. HL-60 cells exhibit increased adherence following differentiation toward either the monocytic or granulocytic pathways [131]. When HL-60 cells have been treated with PMA, they have been shown to exhibit morphologic changes that are characteristic of monocytic cells, including the appearance of pseudopodia, cerebriform nuclei, and the disappearance of azurophilic granules. However, they fail to produce secondary granules that are typical of mature cells indicating incomplete maturation [136]. Following chemically induced monocytic differentiation, increased production of acid phosphatase, β-glucuronidase, and myeloperoxidase has been observed [137]. Thus, the HL-60 cell line exhibits characteristics of an undifferentiated myeloid progenitor. Because of its ability to differentiate toward both granulocytic and monocytic cell types, HL-60 cells are considered a model for cells of the myelomonocytic lineage.

These cells have been widely used in studies on HIV-1 infection. This is because of their ability to be infected in an unactivated state as well as because of the development of the OM-10.1 cell, a clonally derived cell line from HIV-1–infected HL-60 promyelocytes which harbor a single integrated provirus that is silent until activated [138]. In the beginning of the epidemic, a number of studies were conducted with the HL-60 and OM-10.1 cells to determine and characterize the viral infection and replication dynamics within cells of this lineage [138–143]. These cells have been shown to retain CD4, CXCR4, and CCR5 expression and retain CD4 expression unless viral replication is active [138]. Given this observation, the HL-60 and OM-10.1 cell lines have been used in several studies that simply aim at examining the levels of CD4, CXCR4, and CCR5 or other surface markers under various cellular physiological conditions and drug treatments [138, 144–159]. These cells have also been used to screen methodologies or drugs that may inhibit HIV-1 infection or reduce transcriptional activation of the virus [117, 160–173]. These cell lines have also been used in studies of drug toxicity, permeability, and/or effects on cellular activation and differentiation to gain an understanding of what specific drugs might do to cells in the bone marrow [144, 154, 174–183], as well as determining what signaling pathways may play a role or become dysregulated [184–189]. Additionally, other studies have been completed that utilize these cells to examine the role that distinct viral determinants as well as specific host factors have on cellular tropism, cellular differentiation, and cytopathology [190–193]. They have also been used in examining the role of CDK9 and characterizing its function based on known interactions with Tat [166] as well as how Nef manipulates intracellular Ca(2+) stores through SH3-mediated interactions in myelomonocytic cells [194].

Because of the more recent interest in HIV-1 latency, the OM-10.1 cell line has been used to understand drugs that may activate latent viral reservoirs for shock and kill or kick and kill type therapeutics. Some specific examples include a small molecule activator of protein phosphatase-1 (SMAPP-1) [195], NCH-51 [196], hybrid liposomes (HL) composed of dimyristoylphosphatidylcholine (DMPC) and polyoxyethylene alkyl [197], or contact with T cells [198]. Additionally, these cells have been used to characterize the mechanisms involved in maintaining HIV-1 latency [199]. The integrated provirus in these cells seems to be latent due to a transcriptional control mechanism and can be induced by TNF-α, suggesting a potential NF-κB-mediated control [200].

9.4. U-937 and THP-1

U-937 cells are an immature monocytic cell line derived from the pleural effusion of a patient with histiocytic lymphoma [201]. U-937 cells exhibit the morphologic and histochemical characteristics of monoblastic cells, including the expression of ²-glucuronidase and the release of lysozyme into the culture [201, 202]. Only a small percentage of undifferentiated U-937 cells are phagocytic. Furthermore, U-937 cells lack the ability to kill cells expressing foreign antigen presented by MHC class I [203, 204]. U-937 cell lines exhibit characteristics of monoblastic cells in their undifferentiated state, and can be induced to differentiate toward a more mature macrophagic cellular phenotype by a number of chemical agents. PMA can induce differentiation of U-937 cells toward a more mature monocytic phenotype [205, 206]. Differentiated U-937 cells have increased adherence and ramification, along with greater phagocytic activity and the induction of lysozyme and nonspecific esterase activity [206, 207]. Other chemical agents can also be used to induce macrophage differentiation of U-937 cells. Treatment with retinoic acid or 1-25 dihydroxyvitamin D_3 can induce the differentiation of U-937 cells. Like the HL-60 cell line, a U-937 cell line carrying integrated HIV-1 proviral DNA has been constructed with the integrated viral genome in a quiescent configuration that has been shown to be capable of being activated into a transcriptionally active state capable of driving the production of infectious virus. This cell line was termed U1 [208]. Like with HL-60, the U-937 cell line has been used in several types of experiments including experiments to examine what is needed to reactivate the integrated virus [209–214] and most recently in using CRISPR/cas9 technology to excise HIV out of cells as a potential "cure" strategy [215].

THP-1 cells are a monocytic cell line derived from the peripheral blood of a 1-year old male patient who had acute monocytic leukemia [216]. The difference between THP-1 cells and U-937 cells is the origin and maturation stage of both cell lines. U-937 cells are of tissue origin and are therefore at a more mature stage. THP-1 cells are derived from a blood leukemia which represents a less mature stage. There is extensive literature describing the use of vitamin D3 or PMA to differentiate THP-1 cells into macrophages [216]. Recent literature has determined a protocol for PMA that seems to be the most effective to allow differentiation of THP-1 monocytes into macrophages [217]. Interestingly, comparing peripheral blood mononuclear cells (PBMC) monocytes and THP-1 cells has uncovered slight variations in their response to various stimuli. Upon stimulation with Lipopolysaccharide (LPS), PBMC monocytes produce a greater amount of proinflammatory cytokines such as, TNF-α, IL-6, and IL-8 compared to THP-1 cells [218]. These variations in response become much more similar when PBMC and THP-1 monocytes are differentiated into macrophages [219]. Interestingand important for several lines of experimentation, THP-1 cells can be polarized to the M1 or M2 phenotype depending on the stimuli provided.

Due to the differentiation state of U-937 and THP-1 cells, they have been used very widely to mimic HIV-1 infection of peripheral blood monocytes. Due to this, we will not review their use in HIV-1 research in depth as this review focused on promyelomonocytic cell systems. However, there have been some recent reviews that have focused more specifically on the peripheral blood monocytes as well as their utility in studies of HIV-1 latency [220–223].

10. Conclusion

Although HIV-1 may not be able to infect CD34$^+$ stem cells, the research described above shows that they are able to infect the more differentiated progenitor cells. As the cells differentiate from the CD34$^+$ stem cell, the HIV-1 receptor and coreceptor profiles become altered and enhance HIV-1 infection. Thus, the virus infects progenitor cells as they differentiate down the myeloid lineage in the BM and in the blood. Research surrounding this line of investigation has come from examining cells from patients as well as through development of derivative cell lines. As described here the KG-1, TF-1, and HL-60 cell lines have all been used to understand at which stage of the myeloid cell lineage HIV-1 may be able to infect. This has resulted in understanding this is restricted primarily by the levels of CD4 and CXCR4 or CCR5 on the cells. Given this it appears that HIV-1 can infect cells as early as the pluripotent myeloid precursor (**Figure 2**). Because of these models there has been extensive work to examine drug toxicities, regulation of HIV-1 infection, and understanding of how HIV-1 may affect hematopoiesis. However, due to ART making HIV-1 infection a more chronic condition and the theory that one of the main reservoirs may involve the myeloid lineage of cells, including the promyelomonocytic cells of the bone marrow. Hence, this cellular compartment has now taken on a renewed interest. This is evident in the use of the OM-10.1 cell line model for mechanistic studies concerning HIV-1 latency as well as testing of latency reactivators on the various cell lines derived from this lineage of cells. It is the role of the myeloid precursor cells during the course of chronic infection that will be one of the major focal points of future research studies. The use of the TF-1 and HL-60 cells especially, will be very useful with respect to answering questions focused on determining when do these cells transverse the vascular endothelium at an increased rate. Do these infected bone marrow–derived cells traffic to end organs? Do they contribute to the increase in activated monocytes observed in the blood that link to HIV-1-associated neurocognitive impairment? Are these promyelomonocytic cells in the bone marrow infected by cell-free HIV-1 or through cell-to-cell contact with other cells? Are the viruses that infect these cells more dependent on CXCR4 or CCR5 and is there genetic variability more related to a reservoir virus that was generated early in infection and has remained or has continually developed over time in infected patients? These are a few questions that these cell lines will help to answer as research in this field advances.

Author details

Michael R. Nonnemacher[1,2,†], Shane Quiterio[1,2,†], Alexander G. Allen[1,2], Anthony R. Mele[1,2], Vanessa Pirrone[1,2] and Brian Wigdahl[1,2,3*]

*Address all correspondence to: bwigdahl@drexelmed.edu

1 Department of Microbiology and Immunology, Drexel University College of Medicine, Philadelphia, USA

2 Center for Molecular Virology and Translational Neuroscience, Institute for Molecular Medicine and Infectious Disease, Drexel University College of Medicine, Philadelphia, USA

3 Sidney Kimmel Cancer Center, Thomas Jefferson University, Philadelphia, USA

† Authors contributed equally

References

[1] Zhao X, Sun NC, Witt MD, Keller M, Niihara Y. Changing pattern of AIDS: a bone marrow study. Am J Clin Pathol. 2004; 121(3): 393–401.

[2] Isgro A, Aiuti A, Leti W, Gramiccioni C, Esposito A, Mezzaroma I, Aiuti F. Immunodysregulation of HIV disease at bone marrow level. Autoimmun Rev. 2005; 4(8): 486–490.

[3] Lee CI, Cowan MJ, Kohn DB, Tarantal AF. Simian immunodeficiency virus infection of hematopoietic stem cells and bone marrow stromal cells. J Acquir Immune Defic Syndr. 2004; 36(1): 553–561.

[4] Moses AV, Williams S, Heneveld ML, Strussenberg J, Rarick M, Loveless M, Bagby G, Nelson JA. Human immunodeficiency virus infection of bone marrow endothelium reduces induction of stromal hematopoietic growth factors. Blood. 1996; 87(3): 919–925.

[5] Bahner I, Kearns K, Coutinho S, Leonard EH, Kohn DB. Infection of human marrow stroma by human immunodeficiency virus-1 (HIV-1) is both required and sufficient for HIV-1-induced hematopoietic suppression in vitro: demonstration by gene modification of primary human stroma. Blood. 1997; 90(5): 1787–1798.

[6] Durand CM, Ghiaur G, Siliciano JD, Rabi SA, Eisele EE, Salgado M, Shan L, Lai JF, Zhang H, Margolick J, Jones RJ, Gallant JE, Ambinder RF, Siliciano RF. HIV-1 DNA is detected in bone marrow populations containing CD4+ T cells but is not found in purified CD34+ hematopoietic progenitor cells in most patients on antiretroviral therapy. J Infect Dis. 2012; 205(6): 1014–1018. DOI: 10.1093/infdis/jir884

[7] Bordoni V, Bibas M, Abbate I, Viola D, Rozera G, Agrati C, Rinaldi A, Amendola A, Ammassari A, Capobianchi MR, Martini F. Bone marrow CD34+ progenitor cells may harbour HIV-DNA even in successfully treated patients. Clin Microbiol Infect. 2015; 21(3): 290 e295–298. DOI: 10.1016/j.cmi.2014.11.003

[8] Moses A, Nelson J, Bagby GCJr. The influence of human immunodeficiency virus-1 on hematopoiesis. Blood. 1998; 91(5): 1479–1495.

[9] Alexaki A, Wigdahl B. HIV-1 infection of bone marrow hematopoietic progenitor cells and their role in trafficking and viral dissemination. PLoS Pathog. 2008; 4(12): e1000215. DOI: 10.1371/journal.ppat.1000215

[10] Steinberg HN, Crumpacker CS, Chatis PA. In vitro suppression of normal human bone marrow progenitor cells by human immunodeficiency virus. J Virol. 1991; 65(4): 1765–1769.

[11] Kitano K, Abboud CN, Ryan DH, Quan SG, Baldwin GC, Golde DW. Macrophage-active colony-stimulating factors enhance human immunodeficiency virus type 1 infection in bone marrow stem cells. Blood. 1991; 77(8): 1699–1705.

[12] Folks TM, Justement J, Kinter A, Schnittman S, Orenstein J, Poli G, Fauci AS. Characterization of a promonocyte clone chronically infected with HIV and inducible by 13-phorbol-12-myristate acetate. J Immunol. 1988; 140(4): 1117–1122.

[13] Ruiz ME, Cicala C, Arthos J, Kinter A, Catanzaro AT, Adelsberger J, Holmes KL, Cohen OJ, Fauci AS. Peripheral blood-derived CD34+ progenitor cells: CXC chemokine receptor 4 and CC chemokine receptor 5 expression and infection by HIV. J Immunol. 1998; 161(8): 4169–4176.

[14] Weichold FF, Zella D, Barabitskaja O, Maciejewski JP, Dunn DE, Sloand EM, Young NS. Neither human immunodeficiency virus-1 (HIV-1) nor HIV-2 infects most-primitive human hematopoietic stem cells as assessed in long-term bone marrow cultures. Blood. 1998; 91(3): 907–915.

[15] Shen H, Cheng T, Preffer FI, Dombkowski D, Tomasson MH, Golan DE, Yang O, Hofmann W, Sodroski JG, Luster AD, Scadden DT. Intrinsic human immunodeficiency virus type 1 resistance of hematopoietic stem cells despite coreceptor expression. J Virol. 1999; 73(1): 728–737.

[16] Zhang Z, Fu J, Zhao Q, He Y, Jin L, Zhang H, Yao J, Zhang L, Wang FS. Differential restoration of myeloid and plasmacytoid dendritic cells in HIV-1-infected children after treatment with highly active antiretroviral therapy. J Immunol. 2006; 176(9): 5644–5651.

[17] Strazza M, Pirrone V, Wigdahl B, Nonnemacher MR. Breaking down the barrier: the effects of HIV-1 on the blood-brain barrier. Brain Res. 2011; 1399: 96–115. DOI: 10.1016/j.brainres.2011.05.015

[18] Atluri VS, Hidalgo M, Samikkannu T, Kurapati KR, Jayant RD, Sagar V, Nair MP. Effect of human immunodeficiency virus on blood-brain barrier integrity and function: an update. Front Cell Neurosci. 2015; 9: 212. DOI: 10.3389/fncel.2015.00212

[19] Bordoni V, Bibas M, Viola D, Sacchi A, Agrati C, Castelli G, Ammassari A, Amendola A, Abbate I, Martini F. Chronic HIV-infected patients show an impaired dendritic cells differentiation of bone marrow CD34(+) cells. J Acquir Immune Defic Syndr. 2013; 64(4): 342–344. DOI: 10.1097/QAI.0b013e3182a40ff7

[20] Weissman IL. Translating stem and progenitor cell biology to the clinic: barriers and opportunities. Science. 2000; 287(5457): 1442–1446.

[21] Gage FH. Mammalian neural stem cells. Science. 2000; 287(5457): 1433–1438.

[22] Williams RJ, Clarke E, Blair A, Evely R, Hale G, Waldmann H, Brookes S, Pamphilon DH. Impact on T-cell depletion and CD34+ cell recovery using humanised CD52 monoclonal antibody (CAMPATH-1H) in BM and PSBC collections; comparison with CAMPATH-1M and CAMPATH-1G. Cytotherapy. 2000; 2(1): 5–14.

[23] Kim H, Whartenby KA, Georgantas RW3rd, Wingard J, Civin CI. Human CD34+ hematopoietic stem/progenitor cells express high levels of FLIP and are resistant to Fas-mediated apoptosis. Stem Cells. 2002; 20(2): 174–182.

[24] Nabors LK, Wang LD, Wagers AJ, Kansas GS. Overlapping roles for endothelial selectins in murine hematopoietic stem/progenitor cell homing to bone marrow. Exp Hematol. 2013; 41(7): 588–596. DOI: 10.1016/j.exphem.2013.02.014

[25] Hardy CL, Minguell JJ. Cellular interactions in hemopoietic progenitor cell homing: a review. Scanning Microsc. 1993; 7(1): 333–341.

[26] Oxley SM, Sackstein R. Detection of an L-selectin ligand on a hematopoietic progenitor cell line. Blood. 1994; 84(10): 3299–3306.

[27] Andrews RG, Bryant EM, Bartelmez SH, Muirhead DY, Knitter GH, Bensinger W, Strong DM, Bernstein ID. CD34+ marrow cells, devoid of T and B lymphocytes, reconstitute stable lymphopoiesis and myelopoiesis in lethally irradiated allogeneic baboons. Blood. 1992; 80(7): 1693–1701.

[28] Aiuti A, Turchetto L, Cota M, Cipponi A, Brambilla A, Arcelloni C, Paroni R, Vicenzi E, Bordignon C, Poli G. Human CD34(+) cells express CXCR4 and its ligand stromal cell-derived factor-1. Implications for infection by T-cell tropic human immunodeficiency virus. Blood. 1999; 94(1): 62–73.

[29] Uchida N, Fleming WH, Alpern EJ, Weissman IL. Heterogeneity of hematopoietic stem cells. Curr Opin Immunol. 1993; 5(2): 177–184.

[30] Zauli G, Re MC, Davis B, Sen L, Visani G, Gugliotta L, Furlini G, La Placa M. Impaired in vitro growth of purified (CD34+) hematopoietic progenitors in human immunodeficiency virus-1 seropositive thrombocytopenic individuals. Blood. 1992; 79(10): 2680–2687.

[31] Lofsness K. Hematography plus: an instructional program in morphologic alterations of blood cells. Minneapolis, MN: Regents of the University of Minnesota; 2000.

[32] Carr JM, Ramshaw HS, Li P, Burrell CJ. CD34+ cells and their derivatives contain mRNA for CD4 and human immunodeficiency virus (HIV) co-receptors and are susceptible to infection with M- and T-tropic HIV. J Gen Virol. 1998; 79 (Pt 1): 71–75.

[33] Reems JA, Torok-Storb B. Cell cycle and functional differences between CD34+/CD38hi and CD34+/38lo human marrow cells after in vitro cytokine exposure. Blood. 1995; 85(6): 1480–1487.

[34] Koka PS, Jamieson BD, Brooks DG, Zack JA. Human immunodeficiency virus type 1-induced hematopoietic inhibition is independent of productive infection of progenitor cells in vivo. J Virol. 1999; 73(11): 9089–9097.

[35] Marandin A, Katz A, Oksenhendler E, Tulliez M, Picard F, Vainchenker W, Louache F. Loss of primitive hematopoietic progenitors in patients with human immunodeficiency virus infection. Blood. 1996; 88(12): 4568–4578.

[36] Metcalf D. Lineage commitment and maturation in hematopoietic cells: the case for extrinsic regulation. Blood. 1998; 92(2): 345–347; discussion 352.

[37] Valledor AF, Borras FE, Cullell-Young M, Celada A. Transcription factors that regulate monocyte/macrophage differentiation. J Leukoc Biol. 1998; 63(4): 405–417.

[38] Bond HM, Bonelli P, Mesuraca M, Agosti V, Masone C, Cuomo C, Nistico A, Tassone P, Tuccillo F, Cecco L, Iacopino L, Barbieri V, Cerra M, Costanzo FS, Morrone G, Venuta S. Identification by differential display of transcripts regulated during hematopoietic differentiation. Stem Cells. 1998; 16(2): 136–143.

[39] Ogawa M. Differentiation and proliferation of hematopoietic stem cells. Blood. 1993; 81(11): 2844–2853.

[40] Yona S, Kim KW, Wolf Y, Mildner A, Varol D, Breker M, Strauss-Ayali D, Viukov S, Guilliams M, Misharin A, Hume DA, Perlman H, Malissen B, Zelzer E, Jung S. Fate mapping reveals origins and dynamics of monocytes and tissue macrophages under homeostasis. Immunity. 2013; 38(1): 79–91. DOI: 10.1016/j.immuni.2012.12.001

[41] Mosser DM, Edwards JP. Exploring the full spectrum of macrophage activation. Nat Rev Immunol. 2008; 8(12): 958–969. DOI: 10.1038/nri2448

[42] Lopez M, Fleisher T, deShazo RD. Use and interpretation of diagnostic immunologic laboratory tests. Jama. 1992; 268(20): 2970–2990.

[43] Hamilton JA. Colony stimulating factors, cytokines and monocyte-macrophages-some controversies. Immunol Today. 1993; 14(1): 18–24.

[44] Fabian I, Shapira E, Gadish M, Kletter Y, Nagler A, Flidel O, Slavin S. Effects of human interleukin 3, macrophage and granulocyte-macrophage colony-stimulating factor on monocyte function following autologous bone marrow transplantation. Leuk Res. 1992; 16(6–7): 703–709.

[45] Young DA, Lowe LD, Clark SC. Comparison of the effects of IL-3, granulocyte-macrophage colony-stimulating factor, and macrophage colony-stimulating factor in supporting monocyte differentiation in culture. Analysis of macrophage antibody-dependent cellular cytotoxicity. J Immunol. 1990; 145(2): 607–615.

[46] Meuret G, Hoffmann G. Monocyte kinetic studies in normal and disease states. Br J Haematol. 1973; 24(3): 275–285.

[47] Meuret G, Batara E, Furste HO. Monocytopoiesis in normal man: pool size, proliferation activity and DNA synthesis time of promonocytes. Acta Haematol. 1975; 54(5): 261–270.

[48] Whitelaw DM, Batho HF. The distribution of monocytes in the rat. Cell Tissue Kinet. 1972; 5(3): 215–225.

[49] Ganz T, Lehrer RI. Defensins. Pharmacol Ther. 1995; 66(2): 191–205.

[50] Naito M. Macrophage heterogeneity in development and differentiation. Arch Histol Cytol. 1993; 56(4): 331–351.

[51] Thomas WE. Brain macrophages: evaluation of microglia and their functions. Brain Res Brain Res Rev. 1992; 17(1): 61–74.

[52] Salmon JK, Armstrong CA, Ansel JC. The skin as an immune organ. West J Med. 1994; 160(2): 146–152.

[53] Weiser B, Burger H, Campbell P, Donelan S, Mladenovic J. HIV type 1 RNA expression in bone marrows of patients with a spectrum of disease. AIDS Res Hum Retroviruses. 1996; 12(16): 1551–1558.

[54] von Laer D, Hufert FT, Fenner TE, Schwander S, Dietrich M, Schmitz H, Kern P. CD34+ hematopoietic progenitor cells are not a major reservoir of the human immunodeficiency virus. Blood. 1990; 76(7): 1281–1286.

[55] Fauci AS. Host factors and the pathogenesis of HIV-induced disease. Nature. 1996; 384(6609): 529–534.

[56] Harbol AW, Liesveld JL, Simpson-Haidaris PJ, Abboud CN. Mechanisms of cytopenia in human immunodeficiency virus infection. Blood Rev. 1994; 8(4): 241–251.

[57] Scadden DT, Zon LI, Groopman JE. Pathophysiology and management of HIV-associated hematologic disorders. Blood. 1989; 74(5): 1455–1463.

[58] Mir N, Costello C, Luckit J, Lindley R. HIV-disease and bone marrow changes: a study of 60 cases. Eur J Haematol. 1989; 42(4): 339–343.

[59] Kulkosky J, Bouhamdan M, Geist A, Nunnari G, Phinney DG, Pomerantz RJ. Pathogenesis of HIV-1 infection within bone marrow cells. Leuk Lymphoma. 2000; 37(5–6): 497–515.

[60] Sun NC, Shapshak P, Lachant NA, Hsu MY, Sieger L, Schmid P, Beall G, Imagawa DT. Bone marrow examination in patients with AIDS and AIDS-related complex (ARC). Morphologic and in situ hybridization studies. Am J Clin Pathol. 1989; 92(5): 589–594.

[61] Calenda V, Sebahoun G, Chermann JC. Modulation of normal human erythropoietic progenitor cells in longterm liquid cultures after HIV-1 infection. AIDS Res Hum Retroviruses. 1992; 8(1): 61–67.

[62] Cen D, Zauli G, Szarnicki R, Davis BR. Effect of different human immunodeficiency virus type-1 (HIV-1) isolates on long-term bone marrow haemopoiesis. Br J Haematol. 1993; 85(3): 596–602.

[63] Davis BR, Zauli G. Effect of human immunodeficiency virus infection on haematopoiesis. Baillieres Clin Haematol. 1995; 8(1): 113–130.

[64] Molina JM, Scadden DT, Byrn R, Dinarello CA, Groopman JE. Production of tumor necrosis factor alpha and interleukin 1 beta by monocytic cells infected with human immunodeficiency virus. J Clin Invest. 1989; 84(3): 733–737.

[65] Sugiura K, Oyaizu N, Pahwa R, Kalyanaraman VS, Pahwa S. Effect of human immunodeficiency virus-1 envelope glycoprotein on in vitro hematopoiesis of umbilical cord blood. Blood. 1992; 80(6): 1463–1469.

[66] Louache F, Henri A, Bettaieb A, Oksenhendler E, Raguin G, Tulliez M, Vainchenker W. Role of human immunodeficiency virus replication in defective in vitro growth of hematopoietic progenitors. Blood. 1992; 80(12): 2991–2999.

[67] Accornero P, Radrizzani M, Delia D, Gerosa F, Kurrle R, Colombo MP. Differential susceptibility to HIV-GP120- sensitized apoptosis in CD4+ T-cell clones with different T-helper phenotypes: role of CD95/CD95L interactions. Blood. 1997; 89(2): 558–569.

[68] Mondal D, Agrawal KC. Effect of HIV type 1 Tat protein on butyric acid-induced differentiation in a hematopoietic progenitor cell line. AIDS Res Hum Retroviruses. 1996; 12(16): 1529–1536.

[69] Calenda V, Graber P, Delamarter JF, Chermann JC. Involvement of HIV nef protein in abnormal hematopoiesis in AIDS: in vitro study on bone marrow progenitor cells. Eur J Haematol. 1994; 52(2): 103–107.

[70] Zauli G, Vitale M, Re MC, Furlini G, Zamai L, Falcieri E, Gibellini D, Visani G, Davis BR, Capitani S, et al. In vitro exposure to human immunodeficiency virus type 1 induces apoptotic cell death of the factor-dependent TF- 1 hematopoietic cell line. Blood. 1994; 83(1): 167–175.

[71] Re MC, Furlini G, Zauli G, La Placa M. Human immunodeficiency virus type 1 (HIV-1) and human hematopoietic progenitor cells. Arch Virol. 1994; 137(1–2): 1–23.

[72] Esser R, Glienke W, von Briesen H, Rubsamen-Waigmann H, Andreesen R. Differential regulation of proinflammatory and hematopoietic cytokines in human macrophages after infection with human immunodeficiency virus. Blood. 1996; 88(9): 3474–3481.

[73] McLemore ML, Grewal S, Liu F, Archambault A, Poursine-Laurent J, Haug J, Link DC. STAT-3 activation is required for normal G-CSF-dependent proliferation and granulocytic differentiation. Immunity. 2001; 14(2): 193–204.

[74] Haq R, Halupa A, Beattie BK, Mason JM, Zanke BW, Barber DL. Regulation of erythropoietin-induced STAT serine phosphorylation by distinct mitogen-activated protein kinases. J Biol Chem. 2002; 277(19): 17359–17366.

[75] Hubel K, Dale DC, Liles WC. Therapeutic use of cytokines to modulate phagocyte function for the treatment of infectious diseases: current status of granulocyte colony-stimulating factor, granulocyte-macrophage colony-stimulating factor, macrophage colony-stimulating factor, and interferon-gamma. J Infect Dis. 2002; 185(10): 1490–1501.

[76] Harrison DE, Astle CM, Lerner C. Number and continuous proliferative pattern of transplanted primitive immunohematopoietic stem cells. Proc Natl Acad Sci U S A. 1988; 85(3): 822–826.

[77] Morrison SJ, Wandycz AM, Akashi K, Globerson A, Weissman IL. The aging of hematopoietic stem cells. Nat Med. 1996; 2(9): 1011–1016.

[78] Youn BS, Mantel C, Broxmeyer HE. Chemokines, chemokine receptors and hematopoiesis. Immunol Rev. 2000; 177: 150–174.

[79] Kumar N. Bone marrow class [Slideshare.net]. 2012. Available from: http://www.slideshare.net/globalsoin/bonemarrow-class. [Accessed: 2016-12-28]

[80] Gill V, Shattock RJ, Freeman AR, Robinson G, Griffin GE, Gordon-Smith EC, Gibson FM. Macrophages are the major target cell for HIV infection in long-term marrow culture and demonstrate dual susceptibility to lymphocytotropic and monocytotropic strains of HIV-1. Br J Haematol. 1996; 93(1): 30–37.

[81] Chelucci C, Hassan HJ, Locardi C, Bulgarini D, Pelosi E, Mariani G, Testa U, Federico M, Valtieri M, Peschle C. In vitro human immunodeficiency virus-1 infection of purified hematopoietic progenitors in single-cell culture. Blood. 1995; 85(5): 1181–1187.

[82] Molina JM, Scadden DT, Sakaguchi M, Fuller B, Woon A, Groopman JE. Lack of evidence for infection of or effect on growth of hematopoietic progenitor cells after in vivo or in vitro exposure to human immunodeficiency virus. Blood. 1990; 76(12): 2476–2482.

[83] Neal TF, Holland HK, Baum CM, Villinger F, Ansari AA, Saral R, Wingard JR, Fleming WH. CD34+ progenitor cells from asymptomatic patients are not a major reservoir for human immunodeficiency virus-1. Blood. 1995; 86(5): 1749–1756.

[84] Davis BR, Schwartz DH, Marx JC, Johnson CE, Berry JM, Lyding J, Merigan TC, Zander A. Absent or rare human immunodeficiency virus infection of bone marrow stem/progenitor cells in vivo. J Virol. 1991; 65(4): 1985–1990.

[85] Kaczmarski RS, Davison F, Blair E, Sutherland S, Moxham J, McManus T, Mufti GJ. Detection of HIV in haemopoietic progenitors. Br J Haematol. 1992; 82(4): 764–769.

[86] Stanley SK, Kessler SW, Justement JS, Schnittman SM, Greenhouse JJ, Brown CC, Musongela L, Musey K, Kapita B, Fauci AS. CD34+ bone marrow cells are infected with HIV in a subset of seropositive individuals. J Immunol. 1992; 149(2): 689–697.

[87] Muench MO, Roncarolo MG, Rosnet O, Birnbaum D, Namikawa R. Colony-forming cells expressing high levels of CD34 are the main targets for granulocyte colony-stimulating factor and macrophage colony-stimulating factor in the human fetal liver. Exp Hematol. 1997; 25(4): 277–287.

[88] Kaushal S, La Russa VF, Gartner S, Kessler S, Perfetto S, Yu Z, Ritchey DW, Xu J, Perera P, Kim J, Reid T, Mayers DL, St Louis D, Mosca JD. Exposure of human CD34+ cells to human immunodeficiency virus type 1 does not influence their expansion and proliferation of hematopoietic progenitors in vitro. Blood. 1996; 88(1): 130–137.

[89] Folks TM, Kessler SW, Orenstein JM, Justement JS, Jaffe ES, Fauci AS. Infection and replication of HIV-1 in purified progenitor cells of normal human bone marrow. Science. 1988; 242(4880): 919–922.

[90] Sloand EM, Young NS, Kumar P, Weichold FF, Sato T, Maciejewski JP. Role of Fas ligand and receptor in the mechanism of T-cell depletion in acquired immunodeficiency syndrome: effect on CD4+ lymphocyte depletion and human immunodeficiency virus replication. Blood. 1997; 89(4): 1357–1363.

[91] De Luca A, Teofili L, Antinori A, Iovino MS, Mencarini P, Visconti E, Tamburrini E, Leone G, Ortona L. Haemopoietic CD34+ progenitor cells are not infected by HIV-1 in vivo but show impaired clonogenesis. Br J Haematol. 1993; 85(1): 20–24.

[92] Zauli G, Vitale M, Gibellini D, Capitani S. Inhibition of purified CD34+ hematopoietic progenitor cells by human immunodeficiency virus 1 or gp120 mediated by endogenous transforming growth factor beta 1. J Exp Med. 1996; 183(1): 99–108.

[93] Re MC, Zauli G, Gibellini D, Furlini G, Ramazzotti E, Monari P, Ranieri S, Capitani S, La Placa M. Uninfected haematopoietic progenitor (CD34+) cells purified from the bone marrow of AIDS patients are committed to apoptotic cell death in culture. AIDS. 1993; 7(8): 1049–1055.

[94] Louache F, Debili N, Marandin A, Coulombel L, Vainchenker W. Expression of CD4 by human hematopoietic progenitors. Blood. 1994; 84(10): 3344–3355.

[95] Deichmann M, Kronenwett R, Haas R. Expression of the human immunodeficiency virus type-1 coreceptors CXCR-4 (fusin, LESTR) and CKR-5 in CD34+ hematopoietic progenitor cells. Blood. 1997; 89(10): 3522–3528.

[96] Schols D, Struyf S, Van Damme J, Este JA, Henson G, De Clercq E. Inhibition of T-tropic HIV strains by selective antagonization of the chemokine receptor CXCR4. J Exp Med. 1997; 186(8): 1383–1388.

[97] Huisman MT, Smit JW, Crommentuyn KM, Zelcer N, Wiltshire HR, Beijnen JH, Schinkel AH. Multidrug resistance protein 2 (MRP2) transports HIV protease inhibitors, and transport can be enhanced by other drugs. AIDS. 2002; 16(17): 2295–2301.

[98] Kim RB, Fromm MF, Wandel C, Leake B, Wood AJ, Roden DM, Wilkinson GR. The drug transporter P-glycoprotein limits oral absorption and brain entry of HIV-1 protease inhibitors. J Clin Invest. 1998; 101(2): 289–294. 10.1172/JCI1269

[99] Hughes ES, Bell JE, Simmonds P. Investigation of the dynamics of the spread of human immunodeficiency virus to brain and other tissues by evolutionary analysis of sequences from the p17gag and env genes. J Virol. 1997; 71(2): 1272–1280.

[100] Lane TE, Buchmeier MJ, Watry DD, Jakubowski DB, Fox HS. Serial passage of microglial SIV results in selection of homogeneous env quasispecies in the brain. Virology. 1995; 212(2): 458–465.

[101] Power C, McArthur JC, Johnson RT, Griffin DE, Glass JD, Perryman S, Chesebro B. Demented and nondemented patients with AIDS differ in brain-derived human immunodeficiency virus type 1 envelope sequences. J Virol. 1994; 68(7): 4643–4649.

[102] Power C, McArthur JC, Johnson RT, Griffin DE, Glass JD, Dewey R, Chesebro B. Distinct HIV-1 env sequences are associated with neurotropism and neurovirulence. Curr Top Microbiol Immunol. 1995; 202: 89–104.

[103] Strizki JM, Albright AV, Sheng H, O'Connor M, Perrin L, Gonzalez-Scarano F. Infection of primary human microglia and monocyte-derived macrophages with human immunodeficiency virus type 1 isolates: evidence of differential tropism. J Virol. 1996; 70(11): 7654–7662.

[104] Gartner S. HIV infection and dementia. Science. 2000; 287(5453): 602–604.

[105] Liu Y, Tang XP, McArthur JC, Scott J, Gartner S. Analysis of human immunodeficiency virus type 1 gp160 sequences from a patient with HIV dementia: evidence for monocyte trafficking into brain. J Neurovirol. 2000; 6 Suppl 1: S70–81.

[106] Williams KC, Corey S, Westmoreland SV, Pauley D, Knight H, deBakker C, Alvarez X, Lackner AA. Perivascular macrophages are the primary cell type productively infected by simian immunodeficiency virus in the brains of macaques: implications for the neuropathogenesis of AIDS. J Exp Med. 2001; 193(8): 905–915.

[107] Fischer-Smith T, Croul S, Sverstiuk AE, Capini C, L'Heureux D, Regulier EG, Richardson MW, Amini S, Morgello S, Khalili K, Rappaport J. CNS invasion by CD14+/CD16+ peripheral blood-derived monocytes in HIV dementia: perivascular accumulation and reservoir of HIV infection. J Neurovirol. 2001; 7(6): 528–541.

[108] Koeffler HP, Golde DW. Acute myelogenous leukemia: a human cell line responsive to colony-stimulating activity. Science. 1978; 200(4346): 1153–1154.

[109] Koeffler HP, Golde DW. Human myeloid leukemia cell lines: a review. Blood. 1980; 56(3): 344–350.

[110] Hulette BC, Rowden G, Ryan CA, Lawson CM, Dawes SM, Ridder GM, Gerberick GF. Cytokine induction of a human acute myelogenous leukemia cell line (KG-1) to a CD1a+ dendritic cell phenotype. Arch Dermatol Res. 2001; 293(3): 147–158.

[111] Hooper WC, Abraham RT, Ashendel CL, Woloschak GE. Differential responsiveness to phorbol esters correlates with differential expression of protein kinase C in KG-1 and KG-1a human myeloid leukemia cells. Biochim Biophys Acta. 1989; 1013(1): 47–54.

[112] Kiss Z, Deli E, Shoji M, Koeffler HP, Pettit GR, Vogler WR, Kuo JF. Differential effects of various protein kinase C activators on protein phosphorylation in human acute myeloblastic leukemia cell line KG-1 and its phorbol ester-resistant subline KG-1a. Cancer Res. 1987; 47(5): 1302–1307.

[113] Vignoli M, Furlini G, Re MC, Ramazzotti E, La Placa M. Modulation of CD4, CXCR-4, and CCR-5 makes human hematopoietic progenitor cell lines infected with human herpesvirus-6 susceptible to human immunodeficiency virus type 1. J Hematother Stem Cell Res. 2000; 9(1): 39–45. DOI: 10.1089/152581600319603

[114] Furlini G, Vignoli M, Ramazzotti E, Re MC, Visani G, La P. A concurrent human herpesvirus-6 infection renders two human hematopoietic progenitor (TF-1 and KG-1) cell lines susceptible to human immunodeficiency virus type-1. Blood. 1996; 87(11): 4737–4745.

[115] Re MC, Vignoli M, Furlini G, Ramazzotti E, Maldini C, La Placa M. In a human lymphomyeloid progenitor cell line (KG-1) HIV-1 gp120 binds to chemokine-receptors CXC-R4 and CCR5, only in the presence of CD4. New Microbiol. 1999; 22(4): 365–368.

[116] Sakagami H, Kishino K, Kobayashi M, Hashimoto K, Iida S, Shimetani A, Nakamura Y, Takahashi K, Ikarashi T, Fukamachi H, Satoh K, Nakashima H, Shimizu T, Takeda K, Watanabe S, Nakamura W. Selective antibacterial and apoptosis-modulating activities of mastic. In Vivo. 2009; 23(2): 215–223.

[117] Erice A, Balfour HHJr, Myers DE, Leske VL, Sannerud KJ, Kuebelbeck V, Irvin JD, Uckun FM. Anti-human immunodeficiency virus type 1 activity of an anti-CD4 immunoconjugate containing pokeweed antiviral protein. Antimicrob Agents Chemother. 1993; 37(4): 835–838.

[118] Kitamura T, Tange T, Terasawa T, Chiba S, Kuwaki T, Miyagawa K, Piao YF, Miyazono K, Urabe A, Takaku F. Establishment and characterization of a unique human cell line that proliferates dependently on GM-CSF, IL-3, or erythropoietin. J Cell Physiol. 1989; 140(2): 323–334. DOI: 10.1002/jcp.1041400219

[119] Kitamura T, Tojo A, Kuwaki T, Chiba S, Miyazono K, Urabe A, Takaku F. Identification and analysis of human erythropoietin receptors on a factor-dependent cell line, TF-1. Blood. 1989; 73(2): 375–380.

[120] Hu X, Moscinski LC, Hill BJ, Chen Q, Wu J, Fisher AB, Zuckerman KS. Characterization of a unique factor independent variant derived from human factor-dependent TF-1 cells: a transformed event. Leuk Res. 1998; 22(9): 817–826.

[121] Cremer I, Vieillard V, De Maeyer E. Interferon-beta-induced human immunodeficiency virus resistance in CD34(+) human hematopoietic progenitor cells: correlation with a down- regulation of CCR-5 expression. Virology. 1999; 253(2): 241–249.

[122] Suzu S, Harada H, Matsumoto T, Okada S. HIV-1 Nef interferes with M-CSF receptor signaling through Hck activation and inhibits M-CSF bioactivities. Blood. 2005; 105(8): 3230–3237. DOI: 10.1182/blood-2004-06-2084

[123] Zhang MY, Harhaj EW, Bell L, Sun SC, Miller BA. Bcl-3 expression and nuclear translocation are induced by granulocyte-macrophage colony-stimulating factor and erythropoietin in proliferating human erythroid precursors. Blood. 1998; 92(4): 1225–1234.

[124] Briggs SD, Scholtz B, Jacque JM, Swingler S, Stevenson M, Smithgall TE. HIV-1 Nef promotes survival of myeloid cells by a Stat3-dependent pathway. J Biol Chem. 2001; 276(27): 25605–25611. DOI: 10.1074/jbc.M103244200

[125] Furlini G, Re MC, Vignoli M, Ramazzotti E, Monari P, La Placa M. The lack of susceptibility to HIV-1 infection in human hematopoietic progenitor TF-1 cell line correlates with the absence of LFA-1 (CD11a) surface adhesion molecule. New Microbiol. 1995; 18(1): 59–67.

[126] Quiterio S, Grant C, Hogan TH, Krebs FC, Wigdahl B. C/EBP- and Tat-mediated activation of the HIV-1 LTR in CD34+ hematopoietic progenitor cells. Biomed Pharmacother. 2003; 57(1): 49–56.

[127] Alexaki A, Quiterio SJ, Liu Y, Irish B, Kilareski E, Nonnemacher MR, Wigdahl B. PMA-induced differentiation of a bone marrow progenitor cell line activates HIV-1 LTR-driven transcription. DNA Cell Biol. 2007; 26(6): 387–394. DOI: 10.1089/dna.2006.0542

[128] Alexaki A, Quiterio SJ, Nonnemacher MR, Shah S, Liu Y, Banerjee A, Li L, Passic S, Pirrone V, Kilareski E, Petrovas C, Wigdahl B. Modeling Bone Marrow Progenitor Cell Differentiation and Susceptibility to HIV-1 Infection. MOJ immunology. 2014; 1(2): 00009–00009. DOI: 10.15406/moji.2014.01.00009

[129] Collins SJ, Gallo RC, Gallagher RE. Continuous growth and differentiation of human myeloid leukaemic cells in suspension culture. Nature. 1977; 270(5635): 347–349.

[130] Gallagher R, Collins S, Trujillo J, McCredie K, Ahearn M, Tsai S, Metzgar R, Aulakh G, Ting R, Ruscetti F, Gallo R. Characterization of the continuous, differentiating myeloid cell line (HL-60) from a patient with acute promyelocytic leukemia. Blood. 1979; 54(3): 713–733.

[131] Collins SJ, Ruscetti FW, Gallagher RE, Gallo RC. Terminal differentiation of human promyelocytic leukemia cells induced by dimethyl sulfoxide and other polar compounds. Proc Natl Acad Sci U S A. 1978; 75(5): 2458–2462.

[132] Lotem J, Sachs L. Regulation of normal differentiation in mouse and human myeloid leukemic cells by phorbol esters and the mechanism of tumor promotion. Proc Natl Acad Sci U S A. 1979; 76(10): 5158–5162.

[133] Fibach E, Peled T, Treves A, Kornberg A, Rachmilewitz EA. Modulation of the maturation of human leukemic promyelocytes (HL-60) to granulocytes or macrophages. Leuk Res. 1982; 6(6): 781–790.

[134] Dayton ET, Perussia B, Trinchieri G. Correlation between differentiation, expression of monocyte-specific antigens, and cytotoxic functions in human promyelocytic cell lines treated with leukocyte-conditioned medium. J Immunol. 1983; 130(3): 1120–1128.

[135] McCarthy DM, San Miguel JF, Freake HC, Green PM, Zola H, Catovsky D, Goldman JM. 1,25-dihydroxyvitamin D3 inhibits proliferation of human promyelocytic leukaemia (HL60) cells and induces monocyte-macrophage differentiation in HL60 and normal human bone marrow cells. Leuk Res. 1983; 7(1): 51–55.

[136] Newburger PE, Chovaniec ME, Greenberger JS, Cohen HJ. Functional changes in human leukemic cell line HL- 60. A model for myeloid differentiation. J Cell Biol. 1979; 82(2): 315–322.

[137] Rovera G, Santoli D, Damsky C. Human promyelocytic leukemia cells in culture differentiate into macrophagelike cells when treated with a phorbol diester. Proc Natl Acad Sci U S A. 1979; 76(6): 2779–2783.

[138] Butera ST, Perez VL, Wu BY, Nabel GJ, Folks TM. Oscillation of the human immunodeficiency virus surface receptor is regulated by the state of viral activation in a CD4+ cell model of chronic infection. J Virol. 1991; 65(9): 4645–4653.

[139] Ushijima H, Kunisada T, Ami Y, Tsuchie H, Takahashi I, Klocking HP, Muller WE. Characterization of human immunodeficiency virus-1-infected cells of myeloid-monocytic lineage (ML-1, HL-60, THP-1, U-937). J Acquir Immune Defic Syndr. 1992; 5(10): 1001–1004.

[140] Semmel M, Macho A, Morozov V, Coulaud D, Alileche A, Plaisance S, Aguilar J, Jasmin C. Replication of human immunodeficiency virus in HL-60 cells. Res Virol. 1992; 143(4): 249–258.

[141] Ushijima H, Abe T. Human immunodeficiency virus infection in central nervous system and myeloid-monocytic lineage. Acta Paediatr Jpn. 1992; 34(3): 371–376.

[142] Ushijima H, Dairaku M, Honma H, Yamaguchi K, Shimizu H, Tsuchie H, Abe K, Yamamoto A, Hoshino H, Muller WE. Human immunodeficiency virus infection in cells of myeloid-monocytic lineage. Microbiol Immunol. 1991; 35(6): 487–492.

[143] Kitano K, Baldwin GC, Raines MA, Golde DW. Differentiating agents facilitate infection of myeloid leukemia cell lines by monocytotropic HIV-1 strains. Blood. 1990; 76(10): 1980–1988.

[144] Beider K, Begin M, Abraham M, Wald H, Weiss ID, Wald O, Pikarsky E, Zeira E, Eizenberg O, Galun E, Hardan I, Engelhard D, Nagler A, Peled A. CXCR4 antagonist

4F-benzoyl-TN14003 inhibits leukemia and multiple myeloma tumor growth. Exp Hematol. 2011; 39(3): 282–292. DOI: 10.1016/j.exphem.2010.11.010

[145] Zoughlami Y, Voermans C, Brussen K, van Dort KA, Kootstra NA, Maussang D, Smit MJ, Hordijk PL, van Hennik PB. Regulation of CXCR4 conformation by the small GTPase Rac1: implications for HIV infection. Blood. 2012; 119(9): 2024–2032. DOI: 10.1182/blood-2011-06-364828

[146] Beltran JA, Pallur A, Chang SL. HIV-1 gp120 up-regulation of the mu opioid receptor in TPA-differentiated HL- 60 cells. Int Immunopharmacol. 2006; 6(9): 1459–1467. DOI: 10.1016/j.intimp.2006.04.018

[147] Garin A, Pellet P, Deterre P, Debre P, Combadiere C. Cloning and functional characterization of the human fractalkine receptor promoter regions. Biochem J. 2002; 368(Pt 3): 753–760. DOI: 10.1042/BJ20020951

[148] Foti M, Phelouzat MA, Holm A, Rasmusson BJ, Carpentier JL. p56Lck anchors CD4 to distinct microdomains on microvilli. Proc Natl Acad Sci U S A. 2002; 99(4): 2008–2013. DOI: 10.1073/pnas.042689099

[149] Kijowski J, Baj-Krzyworzeka M, Majka M, Reca R, Marquez LA, Christofidou-Solomidou M, Janowska- Wieczorek A, Ratajczak MZ. The SDF-1-CXCR4 axis stimulates VEGF secretion and activates integrins but does not affect proliferation and survival in lymphohematopoietic cells. Stem Cells. 2001; 19(5): 453–466. DOI: 10.1634/stemcells.19-5-453

[150] Gupta SK, Pillarisetti K, Thomas RA, Aiyar N. Pharmacological evidence for complex and multiple site interaction of CXCR4 with SDF-1alpha: implications for development of selective CXCR4 antagonists. Immunol Lett. 2001; 78(1): 29–34.

[151] Di Marzio P, Tse J, Landau NR. Chemokine receptor regulation and HIV type 1 tropism in monocyte-macrophages. AIDS Res Hum Retroviruses. 1998; 14(2): 129–138. DOI: 10.1089/aid.1998.14.129

[152] Horuk R, Hesselgesser J, Zhou Y, Faulds D, Halks-Miller M, Harvey S, Taub D, Samson M, Parmentier M, Rucker J, Doranz BJ, Doms RW. The CC chemokine I-309 inhibits CCR8-dependent infection by diverse HIV-1 strains. J Biol Chem. 1998; 273(1): 386–391.

[153] Roberts BD, Butera ST. Changes in CXC-chemokine receptor-4 expression during HIV-1 replication are independent of CD4 modulations. AIDS. 1997; 11(15): 1886–1888.

[154] Davis CB, Dikic I, Unutmaz D, Hill CM, Arthos J, Siani MA, Thompson DA, Schlessinger J, Littman DR. Signal transduction due to HIV-1 envelope interactions with chemokine receptors CXCR4 or CCR5. J Exp Med. 1997; 186(10): 1793–1798.

[155] Dhawan S, Puri RK, Kumar A, Duplan H, Masson JM, Aggarwal BB. Human immunodeficiency virus-1-tat protein induces the cell surface expression of endothelial leukocyte adhesion molecule-1, vascular cell adhesion molecule-1, and intercellular adhesion molecule-1 in human endothelial cells. Blood. 1997; 90(4): 1535–1544.

[156] Pimentel-Muinos FX, Lopez-Guerrero JA, Fresno M, Alonso MA. CD4 gene transcription is transiently repressed during differentiation of myeloid cells to macrophage-like cells. Eur J Biochem. 1992; 207(1): 321–325.

[157] Schlesinger M, Bar-Shavit Z, Hadar R, Rabinowitz R. Modulation of the expression of CD4 on HL-60 cells by exposure to 1,25-dihydroxyvitamin D3. Immunol Lett. 1989; 22(4): 307–311.

[158] Faltynek CR, Finch LR, Miller P, Overton WR. Treatment with recombinant IFN-gamma decreases cell surface CD4 levels on peripheral blood monocytes and on myelomonocyte cell lines. J Immunol. 1989; 142(2): 500–508.

[159] Firestein GS, Reifler D, Richman D, Gruber HE. Rapid and reversible modulation of T4 (CD4) on monocytoid cells by phorbol myristate acetate: effect on HIV susceptibility. Cell Immunol. 1988; 113(1): 63–69.

[160] Venkataraman N, Cole AL, Ruchala P, Waring AJ, Lehrer RI, Stuchlik O, Pohl J, Cole AM. Reawakening retrocyclins: ancestral human defensins active against HIV-1. PLoS Biol. 2009; 7(4): e95. DOI: 10.1371/journal.pbio.1000095

[161] Imai K, Okamoto T. Transcriptional repression of human immunodeficiency virus type 1 by AP-4. J Biol Chem. 2006; 281(18): 12495–12505. DOI: 10.1074/jbc.M511773200

[162] Ng TB, Lam SK, Fong WP. A homodimeric sporamin-type trypsin inhibitor with antiproliferative, HIV reverse transcriptase-inhibitory and antifungal activities from wampee (Clausena lansium) seeds. Biol Chem. 2003; 384(2): 289–293. DOI: 10.1515/BC.2003.032

[163] Okamoto M, Wang X, Debyser Z, De Clercq E, Baba M. Establishment of an in vitro assay system mimicking human immunodeficiency virus type 1-induced neural cell death and evaluation of inhibitors thereof. J Virol Methods. 2003; 108(2): 195–203.

[164] Suffredini IB, Varella D, de Oliviera AA, Younes RN. In vitro anti-HIV and antitumor evaluation of Amazonian plants belonging to the Apocynaceae family. Phytomedicine. 2002; 9(2): 175. DOI: 10.1078/0944-7113-00109

[165] Kulkosky J, Culnan DM, Roman J, Dornadula G, Schnell M, Boyd MR, Pomerantz RJ. Prostratin: activation of latent HIV-1 expression suggests a potential inductive adjuvant therapy for HAART. Blood. 2001; 98(10): 3006–3015.

[166] Ikezoe T, Daar ES, Hisatake J, Taguchi H, Koeffler HP. HIV-1 protease inhibitors decrease proliferation and induce differentiation of human myelocytic leukemia cells. Blood. 2000; 96(10): 3553–3559.

[167] Critchfield JW, Ho O, Roberts BD, Van Lint C, Verdin E, Butera ST. Isoquinolinesulphonamide derivatives inhibit transcriptional elongation of human immunodeficiency virus type 1 RNA in a promyelocytic model of latency. Antivir Chem Chemother. 1999; 10(5): 275–284.

[168] Critchfield JW, Coligan JE, Folks TM, Butera ST. Casein kinase II is a selective target of HIV-1 transcriptional inhibitors. Proc Natl Acad Sci U S A. 1997; 94(12): 6110–6115.

[169] Butera ST, Roberts BD, Folks TM. Ligand passing by the p75 tumour necrosis factor receptor enhances HIV-1 activation. Cytokine. 1996; 8(10): 745–750. DOI: 10.1006/cyto.1996.0099

[170] Kira T, Hashimoto K, Baba M, Okamoto T, Shigeta S. 2-Glycineamide-5-chlorophenyl 2-pyrryl ketone, a nonbenzodiazepin Tat antagonist, is effective against acute and chronic HIV-1 infections in vitro. Antiviral Res. 1996; 32(2): 55–62.

[171] Xu M, Sharma V, Bryans M, Wilkie NM. Identification of a new member of the MNP transcription factor family in differentiated HL60 cells. Biochem Biophys Res Commun. 1996; 226(2): 488–494. DOI: 10.1006/bbrc.1996.1382

[172] Lee MO, Dawson MI, Picard N, Hobbs PD, Pfahl M. A novel class of retinoid antagonists and their mechanism of action. J Biol Chem. 1996; 271(20): 11897–11903.

[173] Mufson RA, Myers C, Turpin JA, Meltzer M. Phorbol ester reduces constitutive nuclear NF kappa B and inhibits HIV-1 production in mature human monocytic cells. J Leukoc Biol. 1992; 52(6): 637–644.

[174] Yasuno T, Ohe T, Takahashi K, Nakamura S, Mashino T. The human immunodeficiency virus-reverse transcriptase inhibition activity of novel pyridine/pyridinium-type fullerene derivatives. Bioorg Med Chem Lett. 2015; 25(16): 3226–3229. DOI: 10.1016/j.bmcl.2015.05.086

[175] Huang SZ, Zhang XJ, Li XY, Kong LM, Jiang HZ, Ma QY, Liu YQ, Hu JM, Zheng YT, Li Y, Zhou J, Zhao YX. Daphnane-type diterpene esters with cytotoxic and anti-HIV-1 activities from Daphne acutiloba Rehd. Phytochemistry. 2012; 75: 99–107. DOI: 10.1016/j.phytochem.2011.11.013

[176] Yanvarev DV, Shirokova EA, Astapova MV, Shram VI, Kukhanova MK, Skoblov YS. 5'-carbamoylphosphonyl-[6-3H]-AZT as a tool for studying metabolic transformations of the nonradioactive counterpart, an inhibitor of HIV replication. Nucleosides Nucleotides Nucleic Acids. 2007; 26(8–9): 897–900. DOI: 10.1080/15257770701505899

[177] Yanvarev DV, Shirokova EA, Astapova MV, Skoblov YS. AZT 5'-Cholinephosphate as an anti-HIV agent: the study of biochemical properties and metabolic transformations using its 32P-labelled counterpart. Nucleosides Nucleotides Nucleic Acids. 2007; 26(1): 23–36. DOI: 10.1080/15257770601052257

[178] Ikezoe T, Bandobashi K, Yang Y, Takeuchi S, Sekiguchi N, Sakai S, Koeffler HP, Taguchi H. HIV-1 protease inhibitor ritonavir potentiates the effect of 1,25-dihydroxyvitamin D3 to induce growth arrest and differentiation of human myeloid leukemia cells via down-regulation of CYP24. Leuk Res. 2006; 30(8): 1005–1011. DOI: 10.1016/j.leukres.2005.12.008

[179] Skoblov Y, Karpenko I, Shirokova E, Popov K, Andronova V, Galegov G, Kukhanova M. Intracellular metabolism and pharmacokinetics of 5'-hydrogenphosphonate of 3'-azido-2',3'-dideoxythymidine, a prodrug of 3'-azido-2',3'-dideoxythymidine. Antiviral Res. 2004; 63(2): 107–113. DOI: 10.1016/j.antiviral.2004.03.001

[180] Nusbaum NJ, Joseph PE. AZT incorporation into mitochondria: study in a human myeloid cell line. DNA Cell Biol. 1996; 15(5): 363–366. DOI: 10.1089/dna.1996.15.363

[181] Nusbaum NJ, Abraham T. Combination antiretroviral chemotherapy: a potential strategy in AIDS-related malignancy. Anticancer Drugs. 1996; 7(1): 109–114.

[182] Balzarini J, Verstuyf A, Hatse S, Goebels J, Sobis H, Vandeputte M, De Clercq E. The human immunodeficiency virus(HIV) inhibitor 9-(2-phosphonylmethoxyethyl)adenine (PMEA) is a strong inducer of differentiation of several tumor cell lines. Int J Cancer. 1995; 61(1): 130–137.

[183] Semmel M, Macho A, Coulaud D, Alileche A, Plaisance S, Aguilar J, Jasmin C. Effect of retinoic acid on HL-60 cells infected with human immunodeficiency virus type 1. Blood. 1994; 84(8): 2480–2488.

[184] Rivas CI, Golde DW, Vera JC, Kolesnick RN. Involvement of the sphingomyelin pathway in autocrine tumor necrosis factor signaling for human immunodeficiency virus production in chronically infected HL-60 cells. Blood. 1994; 83(8): 2191–2197.

[185] Kitano K, Rivas CI, Baldwin GC, Vera JC, Golde DW. Tumor necrosis factor-dependent production of human immunodeficiency virus 1 in chronically infected HL-60 cells. Blood. 1993; 82(9): 2742–2748.

[186] Butera ST, Roberts BD, Leung K, Nabel GJ, Folks TM. Tumor necrosis factor receptor expression and signal transduction in HIV-1-infected cells. AIDS. 1993; 7(7): 911–918.

[187] Franzoso G, Biswas P, Poli G, Carlson LM, Brown KD, Tomita-Yamaguchi M, Fauci AS, Siebenlist UK. A family of serine proteases expressed exclusively in myelo-monocytic cells specifically processes the nuclear factor kappa B subunit p65 in vitro and may impair human immunodeficiency virus replication in these cells. J Exp Med. 1994; 180(4): 1445–1456.

[188] Ushijima H, Kunisada T, Ami Y, Tsuchie H, Takahashi I, Schacke H, Muller WE. Characterization of cells of the myeloid-monocytic lineage (ML-1, HL-60, THP-1, U-937) chronically infected with the human immunodeficiency virus-1. Pathobiology. 1993; 61(3–4): 145–153.

[189] Kunisada T, Sakagami H, Takeda M, Naoe T, Kawazoe Y, Ushijima H, Muller WE, Kitamura T. Effect of lignins on HIV-induced cytopathogenicity and myeloperoxidase activity in human myelogenous leukemic cell lines. Anticancer Res. 1992; 12(6B): 2225–2228.

[190] DiFronzo NL, Pise-Masison CA, Fernandez-Larsson R, Holland CA. Viral determinants of HIV-1 sufficient to extend tropism to macrophages are distinct from the determinants that control the cytopathic phenotype in HL- 60 cells. AIDS. 1997; 11(14): 1681–1688.

[191] Pise-Masison CA, Holland CA. Restricted replication of the HIV-1 T-lymphotropic isolate NL4-3 in HL-60 cells. Virology. 1995; 206(1): 641–645.

[192] Cannon PM, Tenen DG, Feinberg MB, Shin HS, Kim S. Human immunodeficiency virus-1 infection of the human promyelocytic cell line HL-60: high frequency of low-level infection and effect of subsequent cell differentiation. Blood. 1993; 81(2): 437–445.

[193] Pise CA, Newburger PE, Holland CA. Human immunodeficiency virus type 1-infected HL-60 cells are capable of both monocytic and granulocytic differentiation. J Gen Virol. 1992; 73 (Pt 12): 3257–3261. DOI: 10.1099/0022-1317-73-12-3257

[194] Foti M, Cartier L, Piguet V, Lew DP, Carpentier JL, Trono D, Krause KH. The HIV Nef protein alters Ca(2+) signaling in myelomonocytic cells through SH3-mediated protein-protein interactions. J Biol Chem. 1999; 274(49): 34765–34772.

[195] Tyagi M, Iordanskiy S, Ammosova T, Kumari N, Smith K, Breuer D, Ilatovskiy AV, Kont YS, Ivanov A, Uren A, Kovalskyy D, Petukhov M, Kashanchi F, Nekhai S. Reactivation of latent HIV-1 provirus via targeting protein phosphatase-1. Retrovirology. 2015; 12: 63. DOI: 10.1186/s12977-015-0190-4

[196] Victoriano AF, Imai K, Togami H, Ueno T, Asamitsu K, Suzuki T, Miyata N, Ochiai K, Okamoto T. Novel histone deacetylase inhibitor NCH-51 activates latent HIV-1 gene expression. FEBS Lett. 2011; 585(7): 1103–1111. DOI: 10.1016/j.febslet.2011.03.017

[197] Ueoka R, Komizu Y, Matsumoto Y, Zhong Y, Tanaka R, Yamamoto N. Selective inhibitory effects of hybrid liposomes on the growth of HIV type 1-infected cells in vitro. Bioorg Med Chem Lett. 2008; 18(16): 4578–4580. DOI: 10.1016/j.bmcl.2008.07.030

[198] Qi X, Koya Y, Saitoh T, Saitoh Y, Shimizu S, Ohba K, Yamamoto N, Yamaoka S, Yamamoto N. Efficient induction of HIV-1 replication in latently infected cells through contact with CD4+ T cells: involvement of NF-kappaB activation. Virology. 2007; 361(2): 325–334. DOI: 10.1016/j.virol.2006.11.014

[199] Roberts BD, Fang G, Butera ST. Influence of cell cycle on HIV-1 expression differs among various models of chronic infection. Arch Virol. 1997; 142(6): 1087–1099.

[200] Butera ST, Roberts BD, Lam L, Hodge T, Folks TM. Human immunodeficiency virus type 1 RNA expression by four chronically infected cell lines indicates multiple mechanisms of latency. J Virol. 1994; 68(4): 2726–2730.

[201] Sundstrom C, Nilsson K. Establishment and characterization of a human histiocytic lymphoma cell line (U-937). Int J Cancer. 1976; 17(5): 565–577.

[202] Ralph P, Moore MA, Nilsson K. Lysozyme synthesis by established human and murine histiocytic lymphoma cell lines. J Exp Med. 1976; 143(6): 1528–1533.

[203] Larrick JW, Fischer DG, Anderson SJ, Koren HS. Characterization of a human macrophage-like cell line stimulated in vitro: a model of macrophage functions. J Immunol. 1980; 125(1): 6–12.

[204] Ralph P, Harris PE, Punjabi CJ, Welte K, Litcofsky PB, Ho MK, Rubin BY, Moore MA, Springer TA. Lymphokine inducing "terminal differentiation" of the human monoblast leukemia line U937: a role for gamma interferon. Blood. 1983; 62(6): 1169–1175.

[205] Harris PE, Ralph P, Litcofsky P, Moore MA. Distinct activities of interferon-gamma, lymphokine and cytokine differentiation-inducing factors acting on the human monoblastic leukemia cell line U937. Cancer Res. 1985; 45(1): 9–13.

[206] Tsuchiya S, Kobayashi Y, Goto Y, Okumura H, Nakae S, Konno T, Tada K. Induction of maturation in cultured human monocytic leukemia cells by a phorbol diester. Cancer Res. 1982; 42(4): 1530–1536.

[207] Ralph P, Williams N, Moore MA, Litcofsky PB. Induction of antibody-dependent and nonspecific tumor killing in human monocytic leukemia cells by nonlymphocyte factors and phorbol ester. Cell Immunol. 1982; 71(2): 215–223.

[208] Folks TM, Justement J, Kinter A, Dinarello CA, Fauci AS. Cytokine-induced expression of HIV-1 in a chronically infected promonocyte cell line. Science. 1987; 238(4828): 800–802.

[209] Wang X, Sun B, Mbondji C, Biswas S, Zhao J, Hewlett I. Differences in Activation of HIV-1 Replication by Superinfection With HIV-1 and HIV-2 in U1 Cells. J Cell Physiol. 2016. Epub ahead of print. DOI: 10.1002/jcp.25614

[210] Rao P, Ande A, Sinha N, Kumar A, Kumar S. Effects of cigarette smoke condensate on oxidative stress, apoptotic cell death, and HIV replication in human monocytic cells. PLoS One. 2016; 11(5): e0155791. DOI: 10.1371/journal.pone.0155791

[211] Arenaccio C, Anticoli S, Manfredi F, Chiozzini C, Olivetta E, Federico M. Latent HIV-1 is activated by exosomes from cells infected with either replication-competent or defective HIV-1. Retrovirology. 2015; 12: 87. DOI: 10.1186/s12977-015-0216-y

[212] Barquero AA, Davola ME, Riva DA, Mersich SE, Alche LE. Naturally occurring compounds elicit HIV-1 replication in chronically infected promonocytic cells. BioMed Res Int. 2014; 2014: 989101. DOI: 10.1155/2014/989101

[213] Rasmussen TA, Schmeltz Sogaard O, Brinkmann C, Wightman F, Lewin SR, Melchjorsen J, Dinarello C, Ostergaard L, Tolstrup M. Comparison of HDAC inhibitors in clinical development: effect on HIV production in latently infected cells and T-cell activation. Hum Vaccin Immunother. 2013; 9(5): 993–1001. DOI: 10.4161/hv.23800

[214] Palmisano I, Della Chiara G, D'Ambrosio RL, Huichalaf C, Brambilla P, Corbetta S, Riba M, Piccirillo R, Valente S, Casari G, Mai A, Martinelli Boneschi F, Gabellini D, Poli G, Schiaffino MV. Amino acid starvation induces reactivation of silenced transgenes and latent HIV-1 provirus via down-regulation of histone deacetylase 4 (HDAC4). Proc Natl Acad Sci U S A. 2012; 109(34): E2284–2293. DOI: 10.1073/pnas.1202174109

[215] Hu W, Kaminski R, Yang F, Zhang Y, Cosentino L, Li F, Luo B, Alvarez-Carbonell D, Garcia-Mesa Y, Karn J, Mo X, Khalili K. RNA-directed gene editing specifically eradicates latent and prevents new HIV-1 infection. Proc Natl Acad Sci U S A. 2014; 111(31): 11461–11466. DOI: 10.1073/pnas.1405186111

[216] Chanput W, Mes JJ, Wichers HJ. THP-1 cell line: an in vitro cell model for immune modulation approach. Int Immunopharmacol. 2014; 23(1): 37–45. DOI: 10.1016/j.intimp.2014.08.002

[217] Lund ME, To J, O'Brien BA, Donnelly S. The choice of phorbol 12-myristate 13-acetate differentiation protocol influences the response of THP-1 macrophages to a pro-inflammatory stimulus. J Immunol Methods. 2016; 430: 64–70. DOI: 10.1016/j.jim.2016.01.012

[218] Schildberger A, Rossmanith E, Eichhorn T, Strassl K, Weber V. Monocytes, peripheral blood mononuclear cells, and THP-1 cells exhibit different cytokine expression patterns following stimulation with lipopolysaccharide. Mediators Inflamm. 2013; 2013: 697972. DOI: 10.1155/2013/697972

[219] Sharif O, Bolshakov VN, Raines S, Newham P, Perkins ND. Transcriptional profiling of the LPS induced NF-kappaB response in macrophages. BMC Immunol. 2007; 8: 1. DOI: 10.1186/1471-2172-8-1

[220] Cassol E, Alfano M, Biswas P, Poli G. Monocyte-derived macrophages and myeloid cell lines as targets of HIV-1 replication and persistence. J Leukoc Biol. 2006; 80(5): 1018–1030. DOI: 10.1189/jlb.0306150

[221] Planelles V, Wolschendorf F, Kutsch O. Facts and fiction: cellular models for high throughput screening for HIV- 1 reactivating drugs. Curr HIV Res. 2011; 9(8): 568–578.

[222] Watters SA, Mlcochova P, Gupta RK. Macrophages: the neglected barrier to eradication. Curr Opin Infect Dis. 2013; 26(6): 561–566. DOI: 10.1097/QCO.0000000000000014

[223] Redel L, Le Douce V, Cherrier T, Marban C, Janossy A, Aunis D, Van Lint C, Rohr O, Schwartz C. HIV-1 regulation of latency in the monocyte-macrophage lineage and in CD4+ T lymphocytes. J Leukoc Biol. 2010; 87(4): 575–588. DOI: 10.1189/jlb.0409264